POST-POLIO SYNDROME

Leonard R. Powers

POST-POLIO SYNDROME

Lauro S. Halstead MD
Gunnar Grimby MD PhD

EDITORS

HANLEY & BELFUS, INC.
Philadelphia

MOSBY
St. Louis • Baltimore • Boston • Chicago
London • Philadelphia • Sydney • Toronto

Publisher: HANLEY & BELFUS, INC.
                        210 South 13th Street
                        Philadelphia, PA 19107
                        (215) 546-7293
                        FAX (215) 790-9330

North American and worldwide sales and distribution:

                        MOSBY
                        11830 Westline Industrial Drive
                        St. Louis, MO 63146

In Canada: Times Mirror Professional Publishing, Ltd.
                        130 Flaska Drive
                        Markham, Ontario L6G 1B8
                        Canada

Library of Congress Cataloging-in-Publication Data

Post-polio syndrome / Lauro S. Halstead. Gunnar Grimby, editors.
    p.   cm.
    Includes bibliographical references and index.
    ISBN 1-56053-117-7
    1. Poliomyelitis—Complications.   I. Halstead, Lauro S., 1936–
    II. Grimby, Gunnar.
    [DNLM: 1. Postpoliomyelitis Syndrome. WC 555 P8571 1994]
    RC180.1.P673 1994
    616.8'35—dc20
    DNLM/DLC
    for Library of Congress   94-42418
                                                              CIP

POST-POLIO SYNDROME   ISBN 1-56053-117-7

Last digit is the print number: 9 8 7 6 5 4 3 2 1

CONTENTS

CONTRIBUTORS

JAMES C. AGRE, MD, PhD
Professor and Chairperson, Department of Rehabilitation Medicine, University of Wisconsin-Madison Medical School, Madison, Wisconsin

JOHN R. BACH, MD
Associate Professor and Vice Chairman, Department of Physical Medicine and Rehabilitation, UMDNJ-New Jersey Medical School, Newark, New Jersey

JÖRGEN BORG, MD, PhD
Associate Professor, Department of Neurology, Karolinska Hospital; Senior Consultant, Department of Clinical Neuroscience, Division of Neurology, Karolinska Institute, Stockholm, Sweden

KRISTIAN BORG, MD, PhD
Associate Professor, Department of Neurology, Karolinska Hospital; Department of Clinical Neuroscience, Division of Neurology, Karolinska Institute, Stockholm, Sweden

MARINOS DALAKAS, MD
Chief, Neuromuscular Diseases Section, National Institute of Neurological Diseases and Stroke, National Institutes of Health, Bethesda, Maryland

STEVEN T. DINSMORE, DO
Assistant Professor of Clinical Medicine, Center for Aging, University of Medicine and Dentistry of New Jersey, School of Osteopathic Medicine, Stratford, New Jersey

LARS EDSTRÖM, MD, PhD
Professor and Head, Department of Neurology, Karolinska Hospital;
Department of Clinical Neuroscience, Division of Neurology, Karolinska
Institute, Stockholm, Sweden

HUGH GREGORY GALLAGHER
Writer/Consultant, Washington, D.C.

ANNE CARRINGTON GAWNE, MD
Associate Director, Post-Polio Program, Department of Rehabilitation
Medicine, National Rehabilitation Hospital, Washington, D.C.

GUNNAR GRIMBY, MD, PhD
Professor of Rehabilitation Medicine, Department of Rehabilitation Medicine,
Sahlgrenska University Hospital, Göteborg University, Göteborg, Sweden

LAURO S. HALSTEAD, MD
Director, Post-Polio Program, National Rehabilitation Hospital; Clinical
Professor, Department of Medicine, Georgetown University School of Medicine,
Washington, D.C.

JANET M. LIECHTY, MSW, LICSW
Social Work Service/Polt-Polio Program, National Rehabilitation Hospital,
Washington, D.C.

BARBARA C. SONIES, PhD
Chief, Speech-Language Pathology Section, Clinical Center, National Institutes
of Health, Bethesda, Maryland

ERIK VALDEMAR STÅLBERG, MD, PhD
Professor of Clinical Neurophysiology, and Head, Department of Clinical
Neurophysiology, University Hospital, Uppsala, Sweden

JAN WEINBERG, MD
Consultant, Department of Neurology, Sodersjukhuset University, Stockholm,
Sweden

ANTHONY J. WINDEBANK, MD
Professor of Neurology, Mayo Medical School; Department of Neurology,
Mayo Clinic and Mayo Foundation, Rochester, Minnesota

202-877-1000   EXT. 1653

102 Erving Street N. W.

Washington D.C 20010

PREFACE

The disorder of post-polio syndrome (PPS) is undoubtedly as old as paralytic polio itself. The term, however, and the recognition of the clinical entity are relatively
recent. The late effects of polio began gaining widespread recognition in the early
1980s, and the term PPS was coined at about the time of the First International
Post-Polio Conference at Warm Springs, Georgia, in May 1984. In the intervening
years, there has been a sharp and continuing increase in the attention given to polio by researchers and clinicians, leading to a more precise definition of PPS, a better understanding of the possible etiologies, and the development and refinement
of rational and effective strategies for its management. In creating this volume, we
have attempted to present some of the exciting new work being done in the pathogenesis of PPS as well as a state-of-the-art discussion of the best ways to manage
the most important and challenging clinical problems of PPS. A section on personal
and psychosocial issues, which previously have not been adequately emphasized,
offers the reader insight into the special physical and psychosocial challenges of living with PPS.

Amidst this burgeoning interest, questions about PPS as a distinct clinical entity remain: there is no pathognomonic test; the symptoms are subjective and fairly
general; and there is no truly distinctive symptom pattern. In addition, the pathogenesis remains elusive. This volume includes discussions of the tantalizing findings that suggest several possible causes, from motor unit dysfunction due to overwork or premature aging, to persistence of polio fragments, to an immunologic
phenomenon. Perhaps, in time, we will discover that PPS is not a single entity and
that, in fact, there are several well-defined clinical and pathologic subgroups.

In the meantime, clinicians and researchers will continue to be faced with the
the ongoing challenge of recognizing and managing patients with PPS within the
bounds of our current understanding. It is hoped that this book will provide both
a useful reference and a practical guide in this important work.

Lauro S. Halstead, MD
Gunnar Grimby, MD, PhD

ix

1

Are there Immunopathologic Changes in Patients with Post-Polio Syndrome?

STEVEN T. DINSMORE, D.O. /
MARINOS C. DALAKAS, M.D.

The mechanism of the post-polio syndrome has not yet been definitively ascertained. Accepted criteria to identify the syndrome include a prior history of paralytic poliomyelitis, a stable period after recovery, a residual deficit of the initial poliomyelitis, and new muscle weakness and sometimes new muscle atrophy. The definitions of post-polio syndrome acknowledge that fatigue and muscle pain are present in the syndrome but that these features need not be present to meet criteria for the syndrome.[14,25,27]

These clinical features began to emerge in increasing numbers of polio survivors 15 to 20 years ago. Since they were unexpected it was not immediately recognized by the medical community that a late-effects syndrome was developing in the polio survivor. As the pathogenesis of the acute poliomyelitis came under further scrutiny, it has become clear that polio survivors are traveling with a diminished motor neuron pool, that the surviving motor neurons are performing at an increased capacity, and that some of these motor neurons may have suffered initial injury. Recognition of these features in the remaining motor neuron pool has resulted in the conclusion that post-polio syndrome is due to regression of terminal nerves with resultant muscle weakness and muscle overuse.[1,14,16,25,27]

There are immunologic abnormalities observed in some post-polio syndrome patients that are not well accounted for by muscle overuse or neuron exhaustion. These dysimmune features are observed in spinal fluid, blood, muscle, and spinal cord.

SERUM ANTIBODY TITERS

BLOOD CHEMISTRY

Patients with PPS usually have normal blood chemistries, blood counts, and sedimentation rates and normal serum immunoglobulins IgG, IgA, IgM. No autoantibodies with frequency higher than the general population are seen. Antipoliovirus IgG is elevated as it is in the balance of the western population.

SERUM POLIOVIRUS IgG ANTIBODY

Since the population at large has been immunized to poliovirus, it is not possible to evaluate antibody titers in a post-polio patient population with the assumption that an absent or low antibody titer is normal. In North America the general population should have a protective level of antibody. Additional confounding variables are the immunization status of acute poliomyelitis survivors. Some survivors were immunized, others may have acquired attenuated virus in the community. In order to determine whether there is abnormal antipoliovirus antibody production there must be a comparison with the levels seen in the general population or in patients with non–polio-related neurologic disease.

These conditions were satisfied in a study performed by Kurent et al., who compared serum and spinal fluid antipolio antibody (serotypes 1,2 and 3) titers of 6 PPS patients to 48 ALS patients and 53 controls with other neuromuscular disease. The ALS patients and neuromuscular disease controls were matched for age, sex, race, and poliomyelitis vaccine exposure with the PPS patients. No significant difference was found in serum poliovirus antibody titers among the three groups.[30]

Monzon and Dalakas have found an increase in serum antipoliovirus IgG in some patients with PPS.[33] Melchers et al. examined serum of 16 PPS patients for the presence of anti-poliovirus IgM antibody and poliovirus RNA. There was no evidence of antipolio IgM antibody or poliovirus RNA.[31]

Illa et al. have presented evidence that anti-GM_1 antibodies may be present in higher than normal titers in PPS. The anti-GM_1 antibody titers were measured in the serum of patients with PPS, acute paralytic poliomyelitis, ALS, autoimmune non-neurologic diseases, and 12 normal controls.[26] There was moderate elevation of anti-GM_1 antibody (up to 1:320 dilution) in 32% of patients with acute polio, 39% of PPS patients, 25% of ALS patients, 33% of patients with autoimmune disease, and 16% of controls. Because GM_1 epitopes are present on the surface of motor neurons, this finding suggests an ongoing response against motor neuron determinants.[26]

T-CELL SUBSETS

Helper/suppressor (CD4/CD8) ratios have not been consistently altered in post-polio syndrome. In 1984 Dalakas reported T-lymphocyte CD4/CD8 ratios in post-polio syndrome patients with new muscle atrophy (PPMA), those with musculoskeletal complaints only, and 3 asymptomatic polio survivors.[16] Seven patients were studied with PPMA and 6 poliomyelitis survivors with musculoskeletal complaints only. The normal CD4/CD8 ratio is reported to be $1.8 \pm .05$ in this series. The asymptomatic survivors all had normal ratios. In the group with musculoskeletal complaints 5 were normal and 1 had an increased CD4/CD8 ratio. Among those with new muscle atrophy, 4 had increased helper/suppressor ratios, 1 had a reduced ratio, and 2 were normal.

The CD4 (helper) and CD8 (suppressor) lymphocyte subsets can be further subdivided by the presence of additional cell surface markers. A CD4 subset of interest is marked by the anti 2H4 monoclonal antibody. This antibody subdivides peripheral blood CD4+ cells into two functionally distinct populations. The CD4+2H4+ subset and CD4+2H4-subset. The CD4+2H4+ subset has been reported to function as the inducer of the T8+ suppressor cells; thus, this is a suppressor-inducer subset.[35] More recently this subset has been designated CD45R+ rather than 2H4+.[38]

Most of the literature to date has held the position that the CD4+ CD45R+ subset is a suppressor-inducer subset. Sanders et al. have proposed that this subset is a naive, or resting, subset of T-lymphocytes that lose expression of CD45R+ and acquire increased expression of other immunologically relevant markers after stimulation with antigen.[38,39] This is supported by the observation that CD45R+ levels decrease on activated T-cells as interleukin 2 (IL-2) receptor levels increase, suggesting that CD4+ CD45R+ has a role in regulation of IL-2 dependent T-cell proliferation.

Ginsberg et al.[21] performed an analysis of multiple T-cell subsets on 34 poliomyelitis survivors and 22 healthy individuals. The poliomyelitis survivors were divided into two groups: one without new symptoms and the second with new muscle weakness. Each of the poliomyelitis subgroups contained 17 patients. There was no difference between any of the groups in the CD4/CD8 (helper/suppressor) ratios. However there were differences in subsets of the CD4 and CD8 lymphocyte populations between the poliomyelitis survivors and controls. The CD45R+ subset of the CD4 population was depleted in both polio populations compared with healthy individuals.

Dinsmore and Dalakas reported a smaller series of 21 patients who were evaluated for recruitment into a trial of prednisone for post-polio syndrome.[17] These patients had T-cell subsets studied. All patients had new muscle weakness but not all had new muscle atrophy. A comparison was made to a group of 10 controls with other neurologic disease. The mean percentage of CD4+2H4+ (CD4+CD45R+) cells present in the total peripheral blood lymphocytes was compared between the two groups. The percentage of CD4+CD45R+ in the control group was 14.9% while the value in those with post-polio syndrome was 8.3%. There was a nonsignificant trend of diminished CD4+CD45R+ in the post-polio syndrome group, p=0.075.

In summary, the total CD4+/CD8+ ratio does not vary from normal in patients symptomatic with poliomyelitis late effects. The reported changes in a small number of patients may be related to methodology or other nonspecific factors (e.g., infection) that could affect these results. The functions of the cell populations defined by immunophenotyping have not been conclusively defined, as noted in the discussion above on the CD4+CD45R+ population. Thus, even if the subsets are abnormal their significance is unclear.

CEREBROSPINAL FLUID ALTERATIONS

Several investigators have evaluated spinal fluid for the presence of immunoglobulin. This has been an indirect method of determining if there is immunologic activity in the central nervous from latent virus activity or a dysimmune disease.

Dalakas et al. reported the presence of oligoclonal bands in the CSF of three patients with post-polio muscular atrophy in 1984.[15] Later in 1986 the same author reported oligoclonal bands in the CSF in 7 of 13 patients examined.[12] Immunofixation assay revealed that the bands were composed of IgG. Poliovirus and measles virus antibody were measured in the serum and spinal fluid. The ratio of serum to spinal fluid antibody titer was measured and there was no evidence of increased viral antibody production in the central nervous system.

In 1991, Sharief et al. identified oligoclonal IgM bands in 21 of 36 patients with post-polio syndrome and in none of 67 control subjects. Intrathecal synthesis of IgM antibody was found in 21 of the patients with post-polio syndrome and none of the control subjects. In addition to the production of IgM, the post-polio patients had significantly higher cerebrospinal fluid levels of interleukin-2 (IL-2) and soluble interleukin-2 receptors than controls. The intrathecal synthesis of IgM antibodies to poliovirus correlated with the cerebrospinal fluid concentrations of IL-2 and soluble IL-2 receptor.[40] These are provocative findings, identifying immunologic activity in the CNS and the production of specific IgM antibodies, but they have not yet been reproduced by other laboratories.

The Sharief study is a powerful argument in the post-polio literature for a role of poliovirus in the late effects of poliomyelitis. However Melchers et al. in 1992 published a report that casts considerable doubt on the hypothesis that poliovirus may be causative in post-polio syndrome.[31] In this investigation, the authors used polymerase chain reaction (PCR) to identify poliovirus RNA in cerebrospinal fluid and serum from patients with the post-polio syndrome. Serum and cerebrospinal fluid samples were also examined for the presence of poliovirus-specific IgM antibodies using an antibody-capture ELISA method. There was no poliovirus RNA or poliovirus-specific IgM found in any specimen. Further studies are needed with adequate controls to examine the validity of these reports.

MUSCLE

One of the central concerns in post-polio syndrome is muscle function. Muscle force production is likely the most important determinant in the performance of polio survivors. Initial injury to the motor neuron pool and late changes in motor neuron behavior result in alteration of the target muscle. Muscle biopsy of patients with post-polio syndrome has provided insight into the long-term effect of an injured and depleted motor neuron pool on working muscle.

Dalakas et al. have proposed dividing post-polio muscles into four clinically defined subsets:[9,13] 1, Muscles originally affected but partially recovered. 2, Muscles originally affected but fully recovered. 3, Muscles originally spared clinically but now newly symptomatic. 4, Asymptomatic post-polio patients.

The group 1 muscles reveal what might be expected in a system with chronically overexpanded and overused motor unit. In these biopsies there is increased connective tissue, variation in fiber size, occasional necrotic fiber, fiber splitting, and internal nuclei, findings that represent secondary myopathic change. There is also chronic neurogenic change consisting of fiber-type grouping, occasional small and scattered angulated fibers, groups of small fibers, and nuclear clumps. In 2 of 5 biopsies there were mild perivascular inflammatory cells as well as interstitial inflammation.

Group 2 had more predominant findings of recent denervation and chronic denervation and reinnervation. These consisted of larger fiber-type groups (up to 170 normal size fibers) and scattered small angulated fibers. Some secondary myopathic features were also present. In 5 of 14 biopsies perivascular or interstitial inflammation without fiber necrosis was present.

Group 3 muscles again had findings of recent denervation and chronic denervation and reinnervation. Secondary myopathic features were absent. However in 6 of 16 biopsies there was interstitial or perivascular inflammation.

Group 4 muscles revealed only fiber-typed grouping of mild to moderate size. There was no evidence of recent denervation or inflammation in muscles from this category.

Common to all of the symptomatic muscles were some specimens that had perivascular or interstitial inflammation. Overall, 40% of the symptomatic post-polio muscles in these studies had inflammatory findings.[8–10] In 2 patients lymphorrhages were noted.[10] In a later study the cell types composing the inflammatory infiltrates were characterized and counted using immunocytochemical methods.[14] The post-polio muscles were compared with muscle biopsies from non-postpoliomyelitis neurologic controls. Again, 40 percent of the post-polio syndrome muscles had a statistically significant increased number of CD8+ endomysially located lymphocytes. There was also a significant increase of macrophages in the muscle of these patients, although not as prominent as the numbers of lymphocytes. In addition a large number of muscle fibers in the post-polio syndrome patients expressed MHC-class I antigen on their surface. This expression was seen even in areas remote from the lymphocytic infiltrate.

VIRUSES IN THE MUSCLE

Two independent groups, Dalakas et al.[10] and Melchers et al.[31] have failed to amplify viruses in the muscles of PPS patients using PCR. In the report by Dalakas, even in the muscle biopsies that had endomysial inflammation, viral RNA could not be detected.

SPINAL CORD

Pezeshkpour and Dalakas have reported long-term changes in the spinal cords of poliomyelitis survivors.[37] Abnormalities have been observed in the spinal cord of patients with prior acute poliomyelitis. Spinal cords from 8 patients have come to pathologic examination. Five of the patients had stable residual neuromuscular deficits in several limbs but no new weakness. Three had typical PPS. The findings in the post-polio patients were compared with non-poliomyelitis controls composed of 10 patients with ALS and 5 with spinocerebellar degeneration.

All patients had abnormal inflammation in the spinal cord compared with non-polio patients. Five had perivascular and 6 had parenchymal inflammation. These inflammatory exudates consisted of lymphocytes and plasma cells and were seen in all the patients, regardless of the presence of new weakness. There was reactive astrocytosis in all patients. Three patients had the additional finding of axonal spheroids and occasional neurons with signs of chromatolysis.

The average life-span of these patients from time of original illness was 20.7 years. The presence of inflammation was unrelated to the presence of new symptoms; however, neuronal atrophy, chromatolysis, axonal spheroids, and active gliosis were more prominent in the patients with new weakness (PPS). These findings are unexpected in patients whose initial illness occurred decades before the examination. In an acute, self-limited viral illness, the inflammation and gliosis would be expected to end within months after the acute infection had ceased. The presence of axonal spheroids is consistent with recent deterioration. These represent a defect in the movement of trophic material from the neuron down the body of the axon and are found predominantly in patients with motor neuron disease who have recent neuronal degeneration.[7,22] These findings differ markedly from those of amyotrophic lateral sclerosis, the prototype of motor neuron disease. In ALS axonal spheroids are infrequent and gliosis is minimal. The inflammation in the spinal cord has now been confirmed by three independent groups.[32,37,42] Our laboratory has also shown B-cell infiltrates, and we are now using in situ PCR to search for the presence of virus.[10]

DISCUSSION

The serologic findings in post-polio syndrome have not been revealing. The high IgM antipolio antibodies found in 6 of 22 patients by Monzon et

Table 1. History of Immunologic Observations in PPS

	Serum	T-cell Subset	CSF	Muscle	Spinal Cord
1979	Kurent et al.[30] ALS/PPS/control. No diff. in serum IgG				
1984		Dalakas et al.[15] No consistent diff. in CD4/CD8 ratio	Dalakas et al.[15] 3/7 PPMA have oligoclonal bands	Dalakas et al.[15] 4/7 PPMA patients have lymphocytic infiltrate, 2 with lymphorrhages	
1986			Dalakas et al.[12] 7/13 PPMA patients had oligoclonal bands	Dalakas et al.[12] 40% of symptomatic muscle had increased lymphocytes and macrophages	
1988					Pezeshkpour & Dalakas[37] 8 spinal cords examined, all had lymphocyte and plasma cell infiltrates. 3 with axonal spheroids.
1989		Ginsberg et al[21] Depleted CD45R+ (suppressor, inducer, or resting T-cell) population			

Year				
1991	Illa et al.[26] Increased anti-GM_1 antibodies in some PPMA		Sharief, et al.[40] intrathecal IgM production, 1 CSF interleukin-2	
1992	Melchers et al[31] No serum IgM Ab to polio or poliovirus RNA	Dinmore & Dalakas:[17] No difference in CD42H4+ (CD45R+) subsets between PPMA & control	Melchers et al:[31] No CSF-IgM or evidence of poliovirus RNA	Melchers: et al:[31] No evidence of poliovirus RNA in muscle
1994	Monzon et al:[33] A trend of elevated IgG and Igm to poliovirus in PPS		Monzon et al:[33] viral RNA in CSF of 4/12 PPMA patients. Muir et al:[36] 3/24 PPS patients had oligoclonal IgM bands in addition to enteroviral RNA	Miller et al:[32] One patient. Perivascular infiltrates of B-lymphocytes. Tresser et al:[42] 9 PPS patients. 5 with microglial and 2 had perivascular inflammatory infiltrates. Chronic inflammatory meningeal infiltrate

al. correlated with these IgM titers found in patients with acute polio and may suggest an active response against a poliovirus.[33] The significance of peripheral blood lymphocyte subset abnormalities reported by Ginsberg[21] is unknown. The identification of CSF oligoclonal bands appears to be reproducible. These have been reported twice by Dalakas.[12,15] Sharief[40] and Muir[36] have both reported IgM bands. These findings imply that abnormal immunologic dysregulation may exist in the central nervous system. The possibility of persistent virus is now gaining momentum in view of new data,[33,36] although further investigation is needed.

Histologic evidence of inflammation in the spinal cord initially reported by Pezeshkpour and Dalakas has now been supported by the two recently presented studies of Miller[32] and Tresser.[42] These findings, like those in muscle, are clear and do not have the potential for methodologic error of antibody and PCR studies. It is uncertain how these inflammatory infiltrates along with the MHC I signaling in muscle are related, if they represent a primary response to antigen stimulus or nonspecific secondary inflammatory changes.

Possibly the underlying process is in the spinal cord alone, producing the histologic alterations and intermittent CSF antibody or cytokine abnormalities.[40] The muscle inflammation and myopathic features may be secondary to direct mechanical or metabolic injury from overwork.[9,23]

In light of the immunologic abnormalities that have been presented, one must consider that these processes are evidence that an autoimmune component has a role in the pathogenesis of PPS. Although the pathophysiology integrating all of these observations remains unclear, it is increasingly difficult to dismiss these findings as artifact, unexplainable, or irrelevant. The constitutional features of fatigue and pain, aside from situations of extreme biomechanical disadvantage, support such a process in addition to motor unit overwork.

Fatigue is one of the most frequent complaints in post-polio syndrome[3–5,24,25] and may precede the onset of other symptoms and signs such as new muscle weakness or atrophy. Of relevance to the present review, several known autoimmune diseases are associated with prominent fatigue, these include systemic lupus erythematosus (SLE), rheumatoid arthritis, and ankylosing spondylitis.[6,29,43] Multiple sclerosis, an illness that also has an autoimmune component, is associated with severe fatigue.[28] Depletion of CD4+CD45R+ lymphocytes as mentioned earlier in PPS has been demonstrated in multiple sclerosis, SLE, and rheumatoid arthritis.[19,34,41] Whether secreted cytokines or lymphockines play a role is only speculative.

PPS AND PREDNISONE

In light of the findings suggesting a possible autoimmune etiology of post-polio syndrome, it was compelling to determine whether an immunomodulating agent would reduce muscle weakness. Glucocorticoids have a major role in the immunotherapy of a wide range of diseases in which inflammation or immunologically mediated phenomena play a predominant pathophysiologic role. Although their precise mechanisms of action for eliciting anti-inflammatory and immunosuppressive effects are not clear, glucocorticoids have been effective in controlling a variety of patients with immune-related neuromuscular diseases.[11,20] We initiated a study at the NIH to determine if the anti-inflammatory and immunosuppressive effects of high-dose prednisone have a beneficial effect on the new muscle weakness of post-polio patients. The doses and schedule of prednisone used were based on the successful programs of administering prednisone in patients with other immune-inflammatory demyelinating polyneuropathies.[11,20]

A total of 17 patients completed a double-blind placebo-controlled study to determine the effectiveness of high-dose prednisone for the treatment of the new weakness in patients with PPS.[18] The age of subjects was restricted to a maximum of 60 years. The mean age of subjects was 49.5 years, range 37 to 60. The patients were randomly assigned to receive prednisone or placebo. The treatment group was given 80 mg of prednisone daily for 4 weeks followed by a tapering dose reduction to 0 mg daily during the next 20 weeks. The design of the dose taper allowed subjects to receive a minimum of 80 mg of prednisone on alternate days for 16 weeks.

Subjects had extremity muscle strength recorded by manual and quantitative muscle testing. Testing was performed at baseline and every 4 weeks after beginning treatment until completion of the study. Manual muscle test (MMT) results were recorded using the MRC scale. Quantitative strength testing was performed using the Tufts Quantitative Neuromuscular Exam (TQNE) with results recorded in kilograms.[2]

Based on preliminary analysis, there was no significant difference between the control and prednisone-treated groups examined by MMT or quantitative muscle strength testing when treatment group was compared with the control at months 3 and 6 of the study. A total of 3 subjects were withdrawn from the study owing to adverse effects of the treatment, two from the prednisone group and one from the placebo group. Treatment with prednisone could not be recommended owing to the absence of significant treatment effect and the occurrence of adverse effects.[18] If the final analysis confirms that prednisone failed to significantly improve the symptoms of post-polio patients, this does not exclude autoimmune dysregulation as a possible cause.

Many other autoimmune conditions such as multiple sclerosis, cases of polymyositis, or chronic inflammatory polyneuropathy (CIDP) also fail to respond to corticosteroids. Further work needs to be done to clarify whether autoimmune dysregulation, if present, plays a role in the cause of post-polio syndrome. Further, genetically determined susceptibility to immune system malfunction that simultaneously predisposes to poliovirus motor neuron attack and an autoimmune disease should be considered. The possibility that early viral-induced injury to muscle or motor neurons triggers a late autoimmune phenomenon needs to be explored. As discussed earlier, persistent virus or persistence of a virus mutation have not been excluded.

The reproducible findings of inflammation in the muscle and spinal cord, the antipolio virus IgM antibodies in the serum, the various serum autoantibodies such as GM_1, and the oligoclonal bands in the CSF are autoimmune features that are not epiphenomena but instead may suggest a complex, unexpected, and poorly understood role in the cause of PPS.

REFERENCES

1. Agre JC, Rodriquez AA, Tafel JA: Late effects of polio: Critical review of the literature on neuromuscular function. Arch Phys Med Rehabil 72:923–931, 1991.

2. Andres P, Hedlund W, Finison L, et al: Quantitative motor asessment in amyotorphic lateral sclerosis. Neurology 36:937–941, 1986.

3. Berlly MG, Strauser WW, Hall KM: Fatigue in post-polio syndrome. Arch Phys Med Rehabil 72:115–118, 1991.

4. Bruno RL, Cohen JM, Galski T, Frick NM: The neuroanatomy of post-polio fatigue. Arch Phys Med Rehabil 75:498–504, 1994.

5. Bruno RL, Frick NM: Stress and "type A" behavior as precipitants of post-polio sequelae. In Halstead LS, Wiechers DO (eds): Research and Clinical Aspects of the Late Effects of Poliomyelitis. White Plains: March of Dimes, 1987.

6. Calin A, Edmunds L, Kennedy G: Fatigue in ankylosing spondylitis—Why is it ignored? J Rheumatol 20:991–995, 1993.

7. Carpenter S: Proximal axonal enlargement in motor neuron disease. Neurology 18:842–851, 1968.

8. Dalakas MC: Morphologic changes in the muscles of patients with postpoliomyelitis new weakness. A histochemical study of 39 muscle biopsies. Muscle Nerve 9:117, 1986.

9. Dalakas MC: Morphologic changes in the muscles of patients with postpoliomyelitis neuromuscular symptoms. Neurology 38:99–104, 1988.

10. Dalakas MC, et al: Pathology and immunopathology of muscle and spinal cord of

patients with the post-polio syndrome. The Post-Polio Syndrome: Advances in Pathogenesis and Treatment. Ann NY Acad Sci (in press).

11. Dalakas MC: Treatment of polymyositis and dermatomyositis with corticosteroids: A first therapeutic approach. In Dalakas MC (ed): Polymyositis and Dermatomyositis. Stoneham, MA, Butterworth 1988; pp 235–253.

12. Dalakas MC, Elder G, Hallet M, et al: A long term follow-up study of patients with post-poliomyelitis neuromuscular symptoms. N Engl J Med 314:959–63, 1986.

13. Dalakas MC, Hallett M: The Post-Polio Syndrome. In Plum F (ed): Advances in Contemporary Neurology. Philadelphia. F. A. Davis 1988, p 51–94.

14. Dalakas M, Illa I: Post-polio syndrome: Concepts in clinical diagnosis, pathogenesis, and etiology. In: Rowland LP: Amyotrophic Lateral Sclerosis and other Motor Neuron Diseases. Adv Neurol 56:495, 1991.

15. Dalakas MC, Sever JL, Fletcher M, et al: Neuromuscular symptoms in patients with old poliomyelitis: Clinical, virological and immunological studies. In Halstead LS, and Wiechers DO (eds): Late Effects of Poliomyelitis. Miami, Symposia Foundation, 1984.

16. Dalakas MC, Sever JL, Madden DL, et al. Late postpoliomyelitis muscular atrophy: clinical, virologic, and immunologic studies. Rev Infect Dis 6(suppl.2):S562–S567, 1984.

17. Dinsmore S, Dalakas MC: Immunogenetic and immunoregulatory factors in patients with the postpolio syndrome (PPS) (Abstract). Neurology 42(4)Suppl:3:230, 1992.

18. Dinsmore ST, Dambrosia J, Dalakas MC: A double blind placebo controlled trial of prednisone for the treatment of the post-polio syndrome (PPS). The Post-Polio Syndrome: Advances in Pathogenesis and Treatment. Ann N Y Acad Sci (in press).

19. Emery P, Gentry KC, Mackay IR, et al: Deficiency of the suppressor inducer subset of T lymphocytes in rheumatoid arthritis. Arthritis Rheum 30(8):849–856, 1987.

20. Engle WK, Dalakas MC: Treatment of neuromuscular diseases. In Wiederholt WC (ed): Therapy for Neurologic Diseases. New York. J. Wiley Sons, Inc. 1982 pp 51–101.

21. Ginsberg AG, Gale MJ, Rose LM, Clark EA: T Cell alterations in late postpoliomyelitis. Arch Neurol 46:497–501, 1989.

22. Griffin JW, Price DL: Proximal axonopathies induced by toxic chemicals. In Spencer PS, Schaumburg HH (eds): Experimental and Clinical Neurotoxicology. Baltimore, Williams & Wilkins, 1980, pp 161–178.

23. Grimby G, Einarsson, G, Hedberg M, Aniansson A: Muscle adaptive changes in post-polio subjects. Scand J Rehab Med 21:19–26, 1989.

24. Halstead LS, Rossi CD: Late effects of polio: Clinical experience with 132 consecutive out-patients. In Halstead LS, Wiechers DO (eds): Research and Clinical Aspects of the Late Effects of Poliomyelitis Miami: Symposia Foundation, 1987 pp 13–26.

25. Halstead LS: Post-polio sequelae: Assessment and differential diagnosis for post-polio syndrome. Orthopedics 14(11):1209–1217, 1991.

26. Illa I, Agboatwalla M, Monzon M, et al: IgM anti-GM_1 ganglioside antibodies in patients with acute paralytic poliomyelitis: Relevance to the post-polio syndrome and other motor neuron diseases. (Abstract) Ann Neurology 30:298, 1991.

27. Jubelt B, Cashman NR: Neurologic manifestations of the post-polio syndrome. Crit Rev Neurobiol 3(3):199–220, 1987.

28. Krupp LB, Alvarez LA, LaRocca NG, Scheinberg LC: Fatigue in multiple sclerosis. Arch Neurol 45:435–437, 1988.

29. Krupp LB, LaRocca NG, Muir J, Steinberg AD: A study of fatigue in systemic lupus erythematosus. J Rheumatol 17:1450–1452, 1990.

30. Kurent JE, Brooks BR, Madden DL, et al: CSF viral antibodies. Evaluation in amyotrophic lateral sclerosis and late-onset postpoliomyelitis progressive muscular atrophy. Arch Neurol 36(5):269–73, 1979.

31. Melchers W, de Visser M, Jongen P, et al: The postpolio syndrome: No evidence for poliovirus persistence. Ann Neurol 32:728–32, 1992.

32. Miller DC: Post-polio syndrome spinal cord pathology: Case report with immunopathology. The Post-Polio Syndrome: Advances in Pathogenesis and Treatment. Ann NY Acad Sci (in press).

33. Monzon M, Dalakas MC: Virological studies in blood, serum and spinal fluid in patients with post-polio syndrome. The Post-Polio Syndrome: Advances in the Pathogenesis and Treatment. Ann NY Acad SCi (in press).

34. Morimoto C, Hafler DA, Weiner HL, et al: Selective loss of the suppressor-inducer T-cell subset in progressive multiple sclerosis: Analysis with anti-2H4 monoclonal antibody. N Engl J Med 316:67–72, 1987.

35. Morimoto C, Letvin N, Distaso JA, et al: The isolation and characterization of the human suppressor inducer T cell subset. J Immunol 134(3):1509–1515, 1985.

36. Muir P, Nicholson F, Sharief MK, et al: Evidence for persistent enterovirus infection of the central nervous system in patients with previous paralytic poliomyelitis and post-polio syndrome. The Post-Polio Syndrome: Advances in Pathogenesis and Treatment. Ann NY Acad Sci (in press).

37. Pezeshkpour GH, Dalakas MC: Long term changes in the spinal cords of patients with old poliomyelitis: Signs of continuous disease activity. Arch Neurol 45:505–508, 1988.

38. Sanders ME, Makgoba MW, Shaw S: Alterations in T cell subsets in multiple sclerosis and other autoimmune diseases (letter). Lancet 1988, p1021.

39. Sanders ME, Makgoba MW, Shaw S: Human naive and memory T cells: Reinterpretation of helper-inducer and suppressor-inducer subsets. Immunol Today 9:195–199, 1988.

40. Sharief MK, Hentges R, Ciardi M: Intrathecal immune response in patients with the post-polio syndrome. N Engl J Med 325:749–55, 1991.

41. Tanaka S, Matsuyama T, Steinberg AD, et al: Antilymphocyte antibodies against CD4+2H4+ cell populations in patients with systemic lupus erythematosus. Arthritis Rheum 32(4):398, 1989.

42. Tresser N, Kaminski HJ, Hogan RE, et al: Pathological analysis of spinal cords from survivors of poliomyelitis. The Post-Polio Syndrome: Advances in Pathogenesis and Treatment. Ann NY Acad Sci (in press).

43. Wysenbeek AJ, Leibovici L, Weinberger A, Guedj D: Fatigue in systemic lupus erythematosus: Prevalence and relation to disease expression. Br J Rheumatol 32:633–635, 1993.

2

Muscle Function, Muscle Structure, and Electrophysiology in a Dynamic Perspective in Late Polio

GUNNAR GRIMBY, MD, PhD / ERIK STÅLBERG, MD

The muscular impairment in patients with a history of polio varies from none to severe. The relationship between the degree of initial involvement and the effect of various compensatory mechanisms determines the clinical picture, which changes dynamically. Early and late recovery after poliomyelitis depend on a number of factors. Clinical improvement that appears within a *few weeks* after the acute phase is probably due to recovery in the excitability of functional, but not degenerated, motor neurons. Degeneration of neurons, causing peripheral denervation, is compensated by collateral sprouting, i.e., by nerve twigs branching off from surviving motor units overlapping with the denervated ones. This is most likely the main factor explaining recovery within the *first 6–12 months*. Another late compensatory process is the increase in size of the muscle fibers. As a result of these processes, normal muscle strength and presumably normal muscle volume can be seen despite a calculated loss exceeding 50% of the number of motor neurons.

Besides the need for a certain muscle volume and, thus, potential for

15

force development, the metabolic adaptation to endurance activity is also a key issue. It is well known that capillarization and the activity of mitochondrial enzymes adapt to a level dependent on the physical activity.[2,13] With immobilization or reduced physical activity, these factors, of basic importance for aerobic capacity and, thus, performance in endurance activities, are reduced. In polio patients with low general physical activity, reduced aerobic muscle capacity may occur, but it is combined with marked muscle fiber hypertrophy, demonstrating different adaptation patterns for resistance and endurance activities.

In this chapter, we first describe the basic morphologic and electrophysiologic adaptations in muscle function and then review the changes that can be seen over time in persons with polio sequelae. By combining data on muscle strength, muscle structure, and electrophysiologic recordings of the size of the motor units, further insight can be obtained on these compensatory processes.

MUSCLE STRENGTH

For strength measurements, the reader should be reminded of the need for objective measurements of muscle strength in polio patients, either by special dynamometers (such as Cybex[9], Kin-Com,[10] and Lido[1]) or by hand-held manual measuring devices (such as Myometer[8]). Good reliability of repeated dynamometer measurements of knee muscles has been reported by Kilfoil and St. Pierre[14] and by Grimby et al.[10] Manual muscle testing does not give reliable information in muscles with strength levels of fair (being able to move the extremity against gravity) or above, as shown already in the 1960s by Beasly[3] and illustrated in chapter 4 by Agre in this book. Isometric measurements are usually quite adequate, as isometric and isokinetic strength values correlate significantly[7] and change in parallel over time.[11]

Muscle strength can be reduced by various degrees and obviously quite differently in different muscle groups, depending on the distribution of the original polio involvement. Whether the dynamics of the compensatory processes differ between muscle groups, however, has not been studied. The stimulus for muscle fiber hypertrophy may vary between muscle groups, depending on their activity pattern.

It is possible to demonstrate a relationship between the perception of new or increased muscle weakness and measurements of reduction in muscle strength. In follow-up studies of persons with poliomyelitis sequelae, it has been possible to demonstrate significant reduction in muscle strength in those who acknowledge new weakness but not in those who do not acknowledge new muscular weakness.[10,11] Thus, in a group of 44 Swedish patients,[11] a 9% (p <0.01) reduction in strength for knee extension at 60°/s angular velocity during a 4–5 year period was demonstrated. When the patients were divided into two groups, the strength reduction was significant (16%, p <0.01) only among those who reported new muscle weakness. As a comparison, the normal age-dependent reduction in muscle strength in the age ranges of 30–70 years (mean age, 53) can be estimated to be around 2–5% during a similar time period and thus not more than about 1% per year.[5,15]

In the following chapter, we use the terms *unstable* and *stable* muscle function for those who acknowledge and do not acknowledge, respectively, new or increased muscle weakness in the tested extremity. Such a division is better than using the post-polio syndrome classification in studies comparing various muscle parameters.

MUSCLE STRUCTURE

Morphological changes in the post-polio muscle are discussed further in chapter 4 in this volume by Borg and Edström. Here, information is given mainly on the adaptive process with changes in fiber size after loss of motor neurons.

Markedly increased muscle fiber areas are seen in the polio-affected muscles,[4,9] provided that muscle strength is only slightly reduced and there is not severe muscle atrophy. According to the report by Grimby and coworkers[9] on the vastus lateralis muscle, mean fiber area was 8×10^3 μm^2 in the post-polio muscles compared to 4.4 and 4.1×10^3 μm^2 for men and women, respectively, in the control groups. There was an increase in type I as well as type II fibers but a somewhat less increase in type IIB fibers. Similar results were found by Borg and coworkers[4] in the tibialis anterior muscle in polio subjects who were excessive users as defined from electromyography (EMG).

In a 4–5-year follow-up study, no systematic changes in mean muscle fiber area could be seen, but when the changes were analyzed in individual polio subjects, certain patterns were noted.[10] Subjects who acknowledged increased muscle weakness (unstable) did not, as a group, show a significant reduction in muscle fiber area. However, some subjects who had average fiber areas close to three times the control values showed a reduction in size during the follow-up period, usually combined with a decrease in muscle strength, but proportionally less. Obviously, compensation by reinnervation could partially compensate for the reduction in fiber size. Other subjects (stable as well as unstable), on the other hand, showed further increase in fiber size during the follow-up period. These findings illustrate the dynamic process in which increased motor unit use due to the parallel loss of motor units can be a stimulus for further fiber hypertrophy, but also indicate that an optimal size for fiber hypertrophy may be reached. The reduction in size of these very large muscle fibers may be caused by several factors, such as basic biological mechanisms leading to reduced capacity to maintain fiber hypertrophy or fiber size reduction due to disease.

NEUROPHYSIOLOGICAL METHODS

A review of the different methods of testing in the post-polio patient is given to explain their differences as well as to highlight the chief parameters measured by each.

SINGLE-FIBER EMG (SFEMG)

The method of SFEMG is described in detail elsewhere.[19] Two parameters are usually measured. One is *fiber density,* a measure of the number of muscle fibers of a motor unit within a hemisphere within a radius of about 300 μm from the small recording electrode. This measure increases with changes in the topography of muscles fibers within the motor unit, typically in cases of reinnervation. It may also increase in myopathy, but other EMG parameters differentiate these two conditions.

The other parameter is *neuromuscular jitter,* an indicator of neuromuscular transmission. When neuromuscular transmission is disturbed, e.g., in myasthenia gravis, the jitter is increased. With more pronounced disturbance, there is also occasional impulse blockings due to impulse failure. Jitter, however, is also increased in conditions with ongoing reinnervation. This is usually due to immaturity of nerve endings and neuromuscular junctions. There may be both pre-synaptic and postsynaptic reasons. Increased jitter and intermittent neuromuscular blocking are seen in some of the recordings from polio patients, but to such a low degree that neuromuscular failure could only explain part of the muscular symptoms.

CONCENTRIC OR MONOPOLAR ELECTRODE EMG (CONVENTIONAL EMG)

In the most commonly used EMG technique, an EMG electrode, with a recording surface somewhat larger than the SFEMG electrode, records from 0.5–2 mm within the motor unit that normally has a diameter of 5–10 mm. The investigation consists of three phases. First, the muscle is studied at rest. Normally, no activity is recorded. Denervated muscle fibers, not yet reinnervated, usually discharge spontaneously, and so-called fibrillation potentials and positive waves are recorded. These are often signs of recent denervation. In the second phase of examination using weak voluntary muscle activation, motor unit potentials (MUPs) are studied regarding various shape parameters. Long-duration and high-amplitude MUPs reflect reinnervation and are typical of a neurogenic disease. Finally, in the third phase, the patient is asked for maximal contraction of the muscle. Normally, a large number of independently firing motor units create a "noise" signal. In cases of a neurogenic condition with loss of some motor units and reinnervation of others, the pattern during maximal contraction shows higher amplitudes of the peaks and overall a less dense signal. All these parameters can be quantitated.

In every patient with polio, at least some muscles show neurogenic changes on EMG, i.e., MUPs with long duration and high amplitudes. Such changes are often found even in muscles that are clinically normal in strength and volume. By complete reinnervation, a full functional restoration can be achieved.

In some muscles denervation activity is seen, usually as fibrillation potentials. This is often due to denervation after recent loss of neurons as an effect of age. Sometimes, this finding may be due to local reasons, such as radiculopathy or nerve entrapment, unrelated to polio (not uncommon in nonpolio patients) or is due to unfavorable situations related to sequelae of polio. If the reason is due to local and definable causes, these should be treated if possible. If no obvious cause is found, the signs of denervation may indicate progressive neurodegeneration, which may lead to muscle symptoms.

MACRO-EMG

Macro-EMG is a relatively new method, described in detail elsewhere.[17,19] It is used to study the total electrical strength of a motor unit. The amplitude of the obtained signal depends on the number and size of muscle fibers in one motor unit. The recording electrode consists of a modified SFEMG electrode with the cannula insulated except for a 15-mm tip. The

SFEMG recording surface is exposed 7.5 mm behind the tip. Recording is made on two channels using a two-channel EMG machine connected to a personal computer for analysis (Intersoft software). On one, the signal from the cannula (using a surface electrode as reference) is recorded and fed to an averager. On the other, the SFEMG recording is obtained between the small surface and the cannula. This signal serves as a trigger for the averaging process. Amplifier filters are set to 5 Hz to 10 kHz and to 500 Hz to 10 kHz for macro and SFEMG, respectively. The electrode is inserted into the voluntarily activated muscle, and a position is sought where an acceptable SFEMG potential is seen. At this moment, the averaging process starts and continues until a smooth baseline and a constant macro MUP is obtained on the "cannula" channel.

ELECTROMYOGRAPHIC FINDINGS

In a recent study[18] of 18 patients with two examinations 4 years apart, macro-EMG recordings from vastus lateralis muscle were used to quantify muscle changes. Muscle biopsies were taken in this muscle, and maximal isokinetic and isometric torque measurements of knee extension were performed. The results are briefly summarized as follows: At the initial evaluation, the macro MUP amplitudes were increased, compared to age-matched controls, by 10 times in the stable group and 16 times in the unstable group, an intergroup difference that is significant (p <0.01). There was no correlation between EMG findings and strength values during the initial examination. Four years later, the strength was unchanged in the stable group but decreased in the unstable, as described earlier, whereas the macro MUP amplitude had increased by 67% and 35% in the stable and unstable groups, respectively. This increase could not be explained by a change in fiber area, which on an average was unchanged.

In two other macro-EMG studies, no increase over time was demonstrated. In one of them,[21] this conclusion was based on the lack of correlation between macro-EMG size and time from acute polio, although the possibility of changes with time was not excluded. In the other study,[16] two examinations were performed 1 year apart with no consistent change in macro MUP.

GENERAL DISCUSSION

The dynamics of late changes after polio are summarized briefly.

FIBER SIZE

Muscle fiber hypertrophy seems to be a characteristic feature of the muscles in polio patients. The upper limit for this compensatory factor is probably reached earlier than that for reinnervation. This is indicated by the fact that during the 4-year follow-up period, there was no further average increase in muscle fiber area in the studied group, whereas the size of the motor unit due to reinnervation continued to increase. Muscle fiber size depends on muscle activity, as already discussed, but also influences muscle strength. Thus, increased activity of motor units as a consequence of the reduction in number of motor units may be a stimulus for muscle fiber hypertrophy. In that way, muscle strength will be better maintained than it would have been without utilization of that compensatory process.

REINNERVATION

As seen from our macro-EMG studies, there is an on-going denervation/reinnervation years after the acute stage of polio. The motor units successively contain increasing numbers of muscle fibers, to a great extent reflecting the degree of reinnervation. Collateral sprouting is highly effective as a compensatory mechanism after denervation. In patients with acute polio more than 20 years ago, the motor unit size due to reinnervation is often 10–15 times the normal size.

There was no correlation between strength and Macro MUP amplitudes in our study.[18] Such a correlation was reported, however, in another study of 10 patients with L5 rhizopathy or history of polio.[20] Lack of these correlations, however, is not surprising. Strength depends on the varying combinations of the number of motor units, fiber size, and the number of muscle fibers. Furthermore, the contractile properties of reinnervating motor units may be abnormal, with less mechanical output for a given electrical signal.[6] Extramuscular factors, such as joints and connective tissue, may also play a functional role, influencing, for example, the degree of maximal muscle activation and force output. The disturbed neuromuscular transmission, typical of reinnervation, could influence the functional output, as earlier reported,[21] although this was not an important factor in our study.

DECOMPENSATION

Decompensation of the muscle changes in late polio occurs during life due to two phenomena. One is the reversion of the factors discussed earlier.

With decreased daily activity and less training, decompensation related to muscle fiber size and oxidative metabolism will occur. The other factor is the continuous loss of motor neurons, as indicated by the increase in macro-EMG changes. This compensatory mechanism may already be utilized more or less completely. In such a situation, further neuronal loss leads to a functional impairment that is proportional to reduction in neurons.

The reinnervation is limited both by central and peripheral factors. The peripheral factors set the limit when a denervated motor unit is no longer overlapping with other motor units, i.e., when all muscle fibers within certain fascicles belong to one motor unit due to previous reinnervation cycles. Overlapping with another motor unit is a prerequisite for reinnervation.

The central factors are related to the status of the motor neuron. In post-polio subjects, the number of muscle fibers losing their innervation with the degeneration of each anterior horn cell is much larger than typically occurs with normal aging, where the motor units usually are only slightly increased in size. This implies a greater strain on reinnervation mechanisms in patients with earlier enlarged motor units who then have additional loss of neurons. Furthermore, the physiological aging process may be exaggerated due to increased demands on the remaining reduced motor neuron pool. For every movement involving weak muscles, a larger portion of the motor neuron pool is utilized to produce the necessary force. In addition, mechanical strains occurring with reduced muscle mass may damage the muscle at a myofibrillar level.

COMBINATION OF FACTORS

Although some statistical characteristics could be found to separate the stable and unstable groups, none of the measured morphological parameters, strength, or neurophysiological findings could be used to predict post-polio syndrome (as defined by Halstead and Rossi[12]) in the individual patient. Most EMG studies have failed to depict EMG changes that may be used to diagnose or predict post-polio syndrome.[21] Even in studies where functional tests concern individual muscles, the EMG changes may be similar in patients with unstable and stable muscle function.

Thus, muscle strength in post-polio patients reflects the dynamic changes in degeneration, compensation, and decompensation. The progressive enlargement of macro-EMG signals, as a compensatory response to loss of neurons, is only one factor in the dynamic change in muscular strength, since the change in strength is the combined effect of the number of available motor neurons, number and size of muscle fibers in each motor unit, neuromuscular transmission, and the mechanical properties of reinnervated muscle fibers. There are a number of possible combinations of denervation-reinnervation and strength that make interpretation of their relationship difficult:

(1) If there is a loss of functioning motor units, not leading to axonal degeneration and therefore not reinnervation, the macro-EMG will not change while strength decreases. This stage of inexcitable neurons may be seen in the acute phase of polio but not later in life.

(2) If reinnervation is successful, but the strength developed by each individual motor unit is decreased compared to normal motor units, macro MUP amplitude increases but strength will still be maintained. It has been demonstrated that reinnervated motor units in amyotrophic lateral sclerosis are weaker than expected from their electrical size as measured with macro-EMG,[6] and our patients may show a similar situation.

(3) Finally, and probably most importantly, reinnervation may compensate for new denervation until a maximal capacity for reinnervation is reached. After this stage, additional loss of motor units cannot be compensated. A continued loss of motor units will then present clinically as a new or accelerating decrease in strength and activity level over time and may, as a result, also be combined with reduced stimulus to maintain the marked fiber hypertrophy.

REFERENCES

1. Agre JJ, Rodriguez AA: Neuromuscular function in polio survivors at one-year follow-up. Arch Phys Med Rehabil 72:11–14, 1991.

2. Andersen P, Henriksson J: Capillary supply of the quadriceps femoris muscle of man: Adaptive response to exercise. J Physiol (Lond) 270:677–690, 1977.

3. Beasley WC: Quantitative muscle testing: Principles and applications for research and clinical services. Arch Phys Med Rehabil 42:398–425, 1961.

4. Borg K, Borg J, Edström L, Grimby L: Effects of excessive use of remaining muscle fibers in prior polio and LV lesion. Muscle Nerve 11:1219–1230, 1988.

5. Borges O: Isometric and isokinetic knee-extension and flexion torque in men and women aged 20–70. Scand J Rehabil Med 16:45–53, 1989.

6. Dengler R, Konstanzer A, et al: Amyotrophic lateral sclerosis: Macro-EMG and twitch forces of single motor units. Muscle Nerve 13:545–550, 1990.

7. Einarsson G, Grimby G, Stålberg E: Electromyographic and morphological functional compensation in late poliomyelitis. Muscle Nerve 13:165–171, 1980.

8. Ernstoff B, Wetterqvist H, Kvist H, Grimby G: The effects of endurance training on individuals with post-poliomyelitis. (In preparation.)

9. Grimby G, Einarsson G, Hedberg M, Aniansson A: Muscle adaptive changes in post-polio subjects. Scand J Rehabil Med 21:19–26, 1989.

10. Grimby G, Hedberg M, Henning G-B: Changes in muscle morphology, strength and enzymes in a four–five-year-follow-up of post-polio subjects. Scand J Rehabil Med 26:121–130, 1994.

11. Grimby G, Thoren-Jönsson A-L: Disability in poliomyelitis sequelae. Phys Ther 74:415–424, 1994.

12. Halstead LS, Rossi CD: Post-polio syndrome: Clinical experience with 132 consecutive outpatients. In Halstead LS, Wiechers DO (eds): Research and Clinical Aspects of the Late Effects of Poliomyelitis. Birth Defects 23(4):13–16, 1987.

13. Henriksson J, Reitman JS: Time course of changes in human skeletal muscle succinate dehydrogenase and cytochrome oxidase activities and maximal oxygen uptake with physical activity and inactivity. Acta Physiol Scand 99:91–97, 1977.

14. Kilfoil M, St Pierre DMM: Reliability of Cybex II isokinetic evaluations of torque in post-poliomyelitis syndrome. Arch Phys Med Rehabil 74:730–735, 1993.

15. Larsson L, Grimby G, Karlsson J: Muscle strength and speed of movement in relation to age and muscle morphology. J Appl Physiol 46:271–281, 1979.

16. Ravits J, Hallet M, et al: Clinical and electromyographic studies of post-poliomyelitis muscular atrophy. Muscle Nerve 13:667–674, 1990.

17. Stålberg E: MACRO EMG, a new recording technique, J Neurol Neurosurg Psychiatry 43:475–482, 1980.

18. Stålberg E, Grimby G: Dynamic electromyography and biopsy changes in a 4-year follow-up study of patients with a history of polio. Muscle Nerve (in press).

19. Stålberg E, Trontelj JV: Single Fiber Electromyography in Healthy and Diseased Muscle. New York, Raven Press, 1994.

20. Tollbäck A, Borg J, Knutsson E: Isokinetic strength, Macro EMG and muscle biopsy of paretic foot dorsiflexors in chronic neurogenic paresis. Scand J Rehabil Med 25:183–187, 1993.

21. Wiechers DO, Hubbel SL: Late changes in the motor unit after acute poliomyelitis. Muscle Nerve 4:524–528, 1981.

3

Muscle Fiber Morphology in Post-Polio Patients

KRISTIAN BORG, MD, PhD /
LARS EDSTRÖM, MD, PhD

Muscle biopsies from patients with a history of poliomyelitis show a wide variety of morphologic changes. The changes are of a neurogenic character and due to damage of the anterior horn cells. However, secondary so-called myopathic changes are relatively frequent. The histopathologic changes have no specific morphologic "marker" to indicate that the patient has had poliomyelitis. The degree of change depends on the degree of involvement of the motor unit by poliomyelitis and varies from mild to end stage; that is, contractile tissue is replaced by fat and connective tissue (Fig. 1).

New or increased weakness and atrophy in skeletal muscle (i.e., late post-polio muscular atrophy [PPMA], as described by Dalakas et al., may suggest that new or increased histopathologic changes may develop in affected muscles decades after the acute infection.[14]

Many polio patients have muscle weakness or develop new weakness, which may lead to a change in the usage pattern of the remaining motor units. This elicits secondary adaptive changes in the muscle fibers.

Muscle biopsy is also of use to differentiate between changes due to poliomyelitis and other unrelated neuromuscular disorders. For example, inclusion body myositis has been described in a patient with prior polio who developed progressive muscle weakness.[1] Among the polio patients of the

25

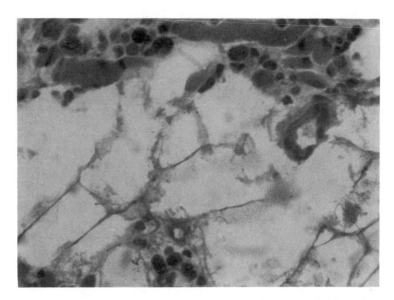

FIGURE 1. Hematoxylin-eosin-stained muscle biopsy from the anterior tibial muscle of a patient with severe muscle weakness due to polio. The muscle fibers (in the upper part of the figure) are atrophic and separated by fat and connective tissue. (Original magnification, ×400.)

authors of the present study, there have been a few with progressive muscle weakness decades after an acute illness with fever. The patients and their relatives attributed the muscle weakness to poliomyelitis. However, clinical findings and muscle biopsy revealed progressive muscular dystrophy.

PATHOLOGY

LIGHT MICROSCOPY

The histopathological changes found in patients with prior poliomyelitis is, as mentioned earlier, mainly of a neurogenic character. In patients with severe muscle weakness there is often extensive fibrosis, and in some patients, there are fatty infiltrates, leading to a serious reduction of contractile tissue (Fig. 1).[5] Such changes are seen in end-stage conditions regardless of whether or not the disorder has a neurogenic or primary myopathic pathogenesis. Muscle fiber changes in less affected patients include type grouping of both type I (slow-twitch) and type II (fast-twitch) fibers, scattered atrophic angulated and rounded fibers (Fig. 2), centrally located nuclei (Fig. 3), fiber splitting (Fig. 3), target fibers, ring fibers, core fibers, moth-eaten fibers, sarcoplasmic bodies, sarcoplasmic masses, and vac-

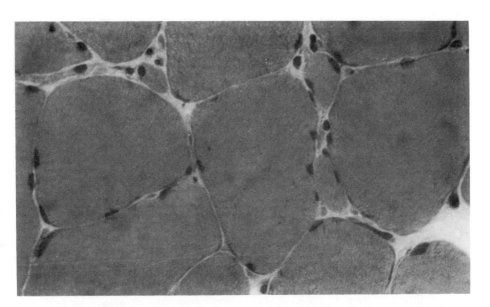

FIGURE 2. Hematoxylin-eosin-stained muscle biopsy from the anterior tibial muscle of a patient with mild muscle weakness due to polio. Note the scattered angulated and rounded atrophic muscle fibers surrounded by muscle fibers of normal size. (Original magnification, ×400.)

uoles.[2,5,8-14,16-18] Rimmed vacuoles (i.e., cytoplasmic vacuoles with a thin rim consisting of basophilic granular material) have also been reported in prior polio patients (Fig. 3).[5]

Infiltrates of inflammatory cells have been reported in some studies,[8-14] and immunological factors or a persistent poliovirus infection has been suggested to play a role in the development of new or increasing muscle weakness. However, inflammatory changes have not been confirmed by other studies,[2,5,17,18,21] and this hypothesis has been regarded with skepticism.

ELECTRON MICROSCOPY

In polio patients with severe weakness, the ultrastructure of the muscle is dominated by widespread fibrosis and a significant reduction of contractile tissue.[5] A myofibrillar disarray (i.e., loss of normally organized myofilaments), replaced by bundles of haphazardly arranged filaments, aggregates of Z-line material resembling rods, and vacuoles, has been described. Other changes in the muscle fibers include large, vesicular, centrally located nuclei; groups of pyknotic, centrally located nuclei; vacuoles; cytoplasmic bodies; and fiber splitting).[5]

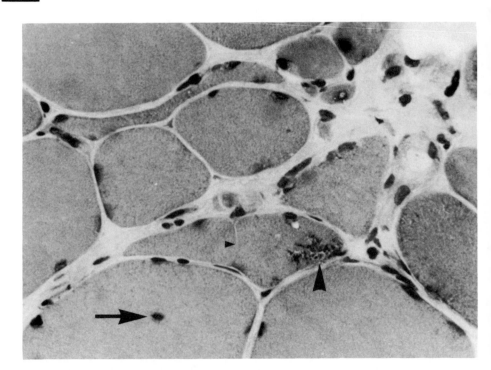

FIGURE 3. Hematoxylin-eosin-stained muscle biopsy from the anterior tibial muscle of a patient with moderate muscle weakness due to polio. Among the muscle fibers with different degrees of atrophy, there is one fiber with a rimmed vacuole (*big arrowhead*) and a splitting phenomenon (*small arrowhead*). An internally located nucleus is indicated by an *arrow.* (Original magnification, ×400.)

In the muscle fibers of patients with a mild degree of weakness, Borg et al. described a well-retained sarcomeric structure with tightly packed, well-aligned myofilaments.[5]

In one patient with prior polio, Schiffer et al. described widened subsarcolemmal areas containing clustered mitochondria and bizarrely shaped giant mitochondria, some of which contained paracrystalline inclusions.[23]

DENERVATION-REINNERVATION

The muscle fiber changes described have been interpreted as being due to ongoing denervation in previously reinnervated motor units.[2,6,9-14] Neurophysiologic studies have given further support for an ongoing denervation-reinnervation process. The cause of the late denervation decades after the acute poliomyelitis is unclear. Furthermore, as of now there are no reliable muscle fiber histopathologic criteria to distinguish between patients with stable weakness and patients with new muscle weakness (i.e., PPMA). Dalakas et al. found an increased amount of small, scattered, angulated muscle fibers in patients with PPMA and suggested that PPMA was due to the death of individual nerve terminals.[10–12] On the other hand, in a study by Cashman et al. there were no morphological differences in muscle biopsies from stable or PPMA patients.[9]

Using macroelectromyography (macro-EMG), Einarsson et al. and Tollbäck et al. showed that the size of the motor unit was increased in patients with prior polio.[15,24] Denervation and reinnervation by means of collateral sprouting should be the main reasons for the increase of the motor unit size. Furthermore, Tollbäck et al. showed that motor unit size was inversely correlated to muscle strength.[24] Thus, loss of motoneurons would be the principal factor behind the decrease in muscle strength in the patients with polio. In the patients studied by Einarsson et al. the minimal degree of motor neuron loss was estimated to be greater than 70%.[15] Grimby et al. described one patient with polio who experienced a decrease in strength during a 2-year follow-up period. Muscle biopsy showed muscle fascicles with hypertrophic type I fibers and fascicles containing only highly atrophic fibers (Fig. 4). Grimby et al. speculated that this was due to denervation in motor units with a previously high degree of reinnervation.[16] Denervation studies of animal experiments give evidence that the perimysium restricts reinnervation.[20] Thus, the increased muscle weakness evident in this patient with polio might be the result of denervation and an inability to sprout over the borders of the muscle fascicles (i.e., an "exhaustion" of the reinnervation capacity).

ADAPTIVE MUSCLE FIBER CHANGES

In an EMG study, Perry et al found muscle overuse during locomotion and suggested that overuse might be the cause of increasing muscular dysfunction in patients with prior polio.[22] In patients with weakness of the anterior tibial muscle due to polio, Borg et al. found an excessive overuse of remaining motor units during walking as determined by EMG.[5] Muscle biopsies in these patients showed almost exclusively type I fibers, which had an increased cross-sectional area (i.e., were hypertrophic) (Fig. 5).[5] In another study, similar findings were seen in the vastus lateralis muscle.[17] In another study by Borg et al., some of the type I fibers contained both

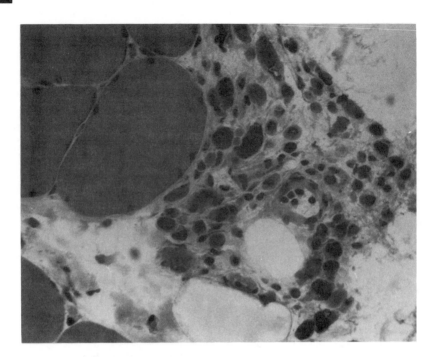

FIGURE 4. Hematoxylin-eosin-stained muscle biopsy from the anterior tibial muscle of a patient with increasing muscle weakness (post-polio muscular atrophy) during a 2-year follow-up period. Note the muscle fibers with normal size and a fascicle with atrophic muscle fibers due to denervation. (Original magnification, ×400.)

slow and fast myosin heavy chains.[4] There was no loss of motor units with high threshold and high axonal conduction velocity normally innervating type II muscle fibers.[3,4] This led Borg et al. to suggest that the lack of type II muscle fibers might be due to a muscle fiber transformation from type II to type I.[4] In a study of isokinetic foot dorsiflexion strength and muscle biopsy in these patients, Tollbäck et al. found that the contractile properties of the overused muscle fibers did not change in parallel with the histochemical fiber type,[25] which is additional support for a muscle fiber–type transformation.

The overused hypertrophic type I muscle fibers had few morphologic and ultrastructural changes,[5] and in a study of cytoskeletal proteins, they exhibited normal cytoskeletal structure.[6] This might indicate that these adaptive muscle fiber changes are adequate to meet the increased demand. Muscle fiber hypertrophy could be expected to compensate for the decrease in muscle strength to a limited extent. On the other hand, low capillary density and decreased oxidative and glycolytic enzyme activity were found in the hypertrophic type I fibers.[7,17,19] These factors may be of im-

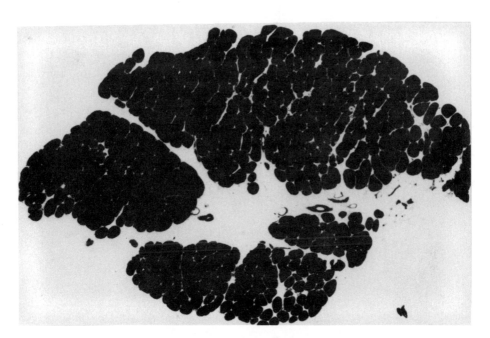

FIGURE 5. Myosin-ATPase (pH 4.3)-stained muscle biopsy from the anterior tibial muscle of a polio patient with muscle weakness and excessive use of remaining motor units during locomotion. Note the total dominance of type I (slow-twitch) muscle fibers. (Original magnification, ×40.)

portance for the development of muscle weakness, fatigue, and muscle pain, which are commonly occurring symptoms in patients with prior poliomyelitis.

ACKNOWLEDGMENTS

This study was supported by grants from the Swedish Medical Research Council (Proj. 3875).

REFERENCES

1. Abarbanel JM, Lichtenfeld Y, Zirkin H, et al: Inclusion body myositis in post-poliomyelitis muscular atrophy. Acta Neurol Scand 78:81–84, 1988.
2. Åbom B, Laursen H, Egsgård H, et al: Late effects of poliomyelitis on muscular function and morphology: A preliminary report. In Halstead LS, Wiechers DO (eds): Research

and Clinical Aspects of the Late Effects of Poliomyelitis. Birth Defects 23(4):223–227, 1987.

3. Borg K, Borg J: Conduction velocity and refractory period of single motor nerve fibres in antecedent poliomyelitis. J Neurol Neurosurg Psychiatry 50:443–446, 1987.

4. Borg K, Borg J, Edström L, et al: Motoneurone firing and isomyosin type of muscle fibres in prior polio. J Neurol Neurosurg Psychiatry 52:1141–1148, 1989.

5. Borg K, Borg J, Edström L, Grimby L: Effects of excessive use of remaining muscle fibers in prior polio and LV lesion. Muscle Nerve 11:1219–1230, 1988.

6. Borg K, Edström L: Prior poliomyelitis: An immunohistochemical study of cytoskeletal proteins and a marker for muscle fibre regeneration in relation to usage of remaining motor units. Acta Neurol Scand 87:128–132, 1993.

7. Borg K, Henriksson J: Prior poliomyelitis-reduced capillary supply and metabolic enzyme content in hypertrophic slow-twitch (type I) muscle fibres. J Neurol Neurosurg Psychiatry 54:236–240, 1991.

8. Brown S, Patten BM: Post-polio syndrome and amyotrophic lateral sclerosis: A relationship more apparent than real. In Halstead LS, Wiechers DO (eds): Research and Clinical Aspects of the Late Effects of Poliomyelitis. Birth Defects 23(4):83–98, 1987.

9. Cashman NR, Maselli R, Wollman RL, et al: Late denervation in patients with antecedent paralytic poliomyelitis. N Engl J Med 317:7–12, 1987.

10. Dalakas MC: Morphologic changes in the muscles of patients with postpoliomyelitis neuromuscular symptoms. Neurology 38:99–104, 1988.

11. Dalakas MC: New neuromuscular symptoms after old polio ("the post-polio syndrome"): Clinical studies and pathogenetic mechanisms. In Halstead LS, Wiechers DO (eds): Research and Clinical Aspects of the Late Effects of Poliomyelitis. Birth Defects 23(4):229–236, 1987.

12. Dalakas MC, Elder G, Hallett M, et al: A long-term follow-up study of patients with post-poliomyelitis neuromuscular symptoms. N Engl J Med 314:959–963, 1986.

13. Dalakas MC, Sever JL, Fletcher M, et al: Neuromuscular symptoms in patients with old poliomyelitis: Clinical, virological and immunological studies. In Halstead LS, Wiechers DO (eds): Late Effects of Poliomyelitis. Miami, Symposia Foundation, 1985, pp 73–89.

14. Dalakas MC, Sever JL, Madden DL, et al: Late postpoliomyelitis muscular atrophy: Clinical, virologic and immunologic studies. Rev Infect Dis 6(Suppl 2):S562–S567, 1984.

15. Einarsson G, Grimby G, Stålberg E: Electromyographic and morphological functional compensation in late poliomyelitis. Muscle Nerve 13:165–171, 1990.

16. Grimby G, Borg J, Borg K, Stålberg E: Postpoliosyndromet—Funktionsnedsättningar hos poliodrabbade. Läkartidningen 89:3179–3182, 1992.

17. Grimby G, Einarsson G: Muscle morphology with special reference to muscle strength in post-polio subjects. In Halstead LS, Wiechers DO (eds): Research and Clinical Aspects of the Late Effects of Poliomyelitis. Birth Defects 23(4):265–274, 1987.

18. Grimby G, Einarsson G, Hedberg M, Aniansson A: Muscle adaptive changes in post-polio subjects. Scand J Rehabil Med 21:19–26, 1989.

19. Henriksson J, Nemeth PM, Borg K, et al: Fibre type-specific enzyme activity profiles. A single fibre study of the effects of chronic stimulation on the rabbit fast-twitch tibialis anterior muscle. In Pette D (ed): The Dynamic State of Muscle Fibres. Berlin, Walter de Gruyter, 1991, pp 385–398.

20. Kugelberg E, Edström L, Abbruzzese M: Mapping of motor units in experimentally reinnervated rat muscle. J Neurol Neurosurg Psychiatry 33:319–329, 1970.

21. Melchers W, de Visser M, Jongen P, et al: The postpolio syndrome: No evidence for poliovirus existence. Ann Neurol 32:728–732, 1992.

22. Perry J, Barnes G, Gronley JK: The postpolio syndrome: An overuse phenomenon. Clin Orthop 233:145–162, 1988.

23. Schiffer D, Palmucci L, Bertolotto A, Monga G: Mitochondrial abnormalities of late motor neuron degeneration following poliomyelitis and other neurogenic muscular atrophies. J Neurol 221:193–201, 1979.

24. Tollbäck A, Borg J, Borg K, Knutsson E: Isokinetic strength, macro EMG and muscle biopsy of paretic foot dorsiflexors in chronic neurogenic paresis. Scand J Rehabil Med 25:183–187, 1993.

25. Tollbäck A, Knutsson E, Borg J, et al: Torque-velocity relation and muscle fibre characteristics of foot dorsiflexors after long-term overuse of residual muscle fibres due to prior polio or L5 root lesion. Scand J Rehabil Med 24:151–156, 1992.

4

Local Muscle and Total Body Fatigue

JAMES C. AGRE, MD, PhD

Fatigue is one of the more common principal reasons given by patients for visits to the internal medicine ambulatory care clinic.[93] For instance, this symptom is more frequently reported than low back pain, arthritis, or head cold. Although fatigue is one of the most frequent complaints in general medical clinics, its specific underlying mechanisms are not well understood, and the ability to objectively and directly measure fatigue in the clinical setting is lacking. As has been discussed by Basmajian, "Fatigue is a complex phenomenon and perhaps a complex of numerous phenomena."[15] Basmajian also pointed out that the fatigue following a strenuous day of effort is probably quite different from the weariness experienced after a long day's routine sedentary work. From our own life experiences, we all know it to be true. Different types of fatigue undoubtedly exist and include emotional fatigue, central nervous system fatigue, "general" fatigue, and peripheral neuromuscular fatigue.[15]

In accordance with the complexity of the nature of fatigue, its definition is somewhat nebulous. According to the American Heritage Dictionary, fatigue is: "1. Physical or mental weariness resulting from exertion. 2. Tiring effort or activity; labor. 3. *Physiol.* The decreased capacity or complete inability of an organism, organ, or part to function normally because of excessive stimulation or prolonged exertion."[12] In a review of metabolic and physiologic factors in fatigue, MacLaren and colleagues provided a physiological definition of muscle fatigue, similar to the aforementioned physiologic definition, namely, the "failure to maintain the required or expected force or power output."[62] The former definition is a reasonable, general definition for fatigue; the latter is as good a definition of local muscle fatigue as is currently available. Neither definition attributes a specific causation to fatigue, which is certainly reasonable at this time, as it reflects our current understanding (actually, lack thereof) of the intricacies and complexities of the fatigue process.

Because relatively little is known about general fatigue, especially as it relates to the post-polio phenomenon, this chapter focuses primarily on muscular fatigue. It is also beyond the scope of this chapter to discuss other medically related causes for fatigue, such as anemia or cardiac, respiratory/pulmonary, or endocrinologic diseases.

CENTRAL AND PERIPHERAL SOURCES OF MUSCULAR FATIGUE

Muscular fatigue may have as its origin both central and peripheral sources. The command chain for muscular contraction involves a number of steps from the brain all the way to the actin-myosin cross bridges within the muscle fibers. Figure 1 depicts the command chain for muscular contraction and the major causes for muscular fatigue. Very briefly, central fatigue may occur as a result of malfunction of nerve cells or inhibition of voluntary effort. In this regard, the action of the sensory pathways on the reticular formation have been suggested as critical.[13] Peripheral fatigue may occur at three possible sites: the neuromuscular junction and muscle cell membrane (excitation), the calcium release mechanism (activation), and the sliding filaments (contractile processes) (Fig. 1).[62] Two hypotheses have been put forth for the causation of fatigue within the muscle: the accumulation hypothesis, related to the accumulation of metabolities such as H^+, ammonia, and inorganic phosphate, and the exhaustion hypothesis, the depletion of certain metabolities such as adenosine triphosphate, phosphocreatine, and glycogen).[84] It is beyond the scope of this chapter to discuss all of these issues in detail, however, and interested readers are referred to previously published work for greater detail.[13,14,62,84]

POST-POLIO FATIGUE

Several reports have documented that polio survivors complain of a number of new musculoskeletal and neuromuscular symptoms.[10,26,29,31,45–48] Table 1 lists several of the most frequent new health problems and prob-

The Command Chain for Muscular Contraction and the Major Causes of Muscular Fatigue

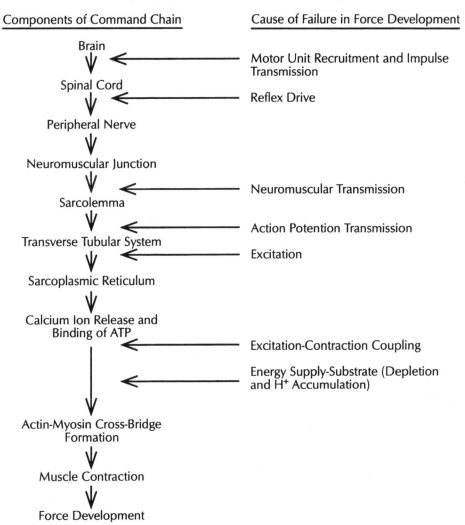

FIGURE 1. The command chain for muscular contraction and major causes of muscular fatigue. (From MacLaren DPM, Gibson H, Parry-Billings M, Edwards RHT: A review of metabolic and physiological factors in fatigue. In Pandolf KB (ed.): Exercise and Sport Sciences Reviews, Vol. 17. Baltimore, Williams & Wilkins, 1989 pp. 29–66, with permission. (Modified from Edwards RHT: Biochemical basis of fatigue. In Knuttgen HG (ed): Biochemistry of Exercise. Champaign, IL, Human Kinetics, 1983, pp 3–28.)

TABLE 1. New Health and ADL Problems

	Percent with Complaint		
	Halstead[45] n = 539	Halstead[46] n = 132	Agre[10] n = 79
Symptom			
Health Problems			
Fatigue	87	89	86
Muscle pain	80	71	86
Joint pain	79	71	77
Weakness			
Previously affected muscles	87	69	80
Previously unaffected muscles	77	50	53
Cold intolerance	–	29	56
Atrophy	–	28	39
ADL Problems			
Walking	85	64	–
Stair climbing	83	61	67
Dressing	62	17	16

ADL = activities of daily living

lems with the activities of daily living (ADL) that are faced by post-polio individuals whether they were seen in a post-polio clinic[10,46] or had responded to a national survey.[45] To be noted, the most prevalent complaint in all three reports is that of fatigue. It should be pointed out that in none of these reports, however, was the term "fatigue" specifically defined, and therefore the underlying basis for the positive response of any individual to this question could not be precisely ascertained.

It is possible that the post-polio individual, in responding to the question about fatigue, was interpreting fatigue to mean one or a combination of the following: emotional fatigue, central nervous system fatigue, "general" fatigue, and/or peripheral neuromuscular fatigue.[15] Only after careful evaluation and interpretation of the fatigue complaint can proper therapeutic measures be taken for an individual patient. It is certainly well-known that some post-polio individuals are experiencing emotional stress or depression,[22,27,40,55] and it is well-known clinically as well as hypothesized for post-polio individuals that both emotional stress and depression can lead a person to feel excessively fatigued.[23]

In a recent small study, fatigue was studied in 12 post-polio patients seen in a post-polio-assessment clinic.[73] It was found that the amount of fatigue these individuals had, as measured by the Fatigue Severity Scale, was over twice that of the nondisabled population and was similar to levels in subjects diagnosed with multiple sclerosis and systemic lupus erythematosus. It has also been reported that, as a part of general fatigue, the individual may experience a pervasive sense of fatigue (such as hitting a wall).[45] From this survey, 43% of individuals reported that they had experienced a phenomenon similar to hitting the wall, and, of that group, 68% acknowledged that the phenomenon occurred on a daily basis. Most commonly, this polio "wall" was experienced in the mid- to late afternoon and it could be ameliorated or aborted by increasing rest time, by napping, or by reducing the overall level of activity during the day.

Three variables found to be associated with the fatigue complaint[45] (hospitalization, ventilator use, and paralysis of all four limbs at the time of the acute poliomyelitis illness) appear to reflect a common underlying variable, namely, severity of the acute poliomyelitis illness. The precise mechanism(s) for this complaint is (are) unknown, but it appears that the underlying cause for "hitting the wall" may be central in origin, as rest and reduction in overall activity appear to be helpful.

Bruno and colleagues hypothesized that the severe, debilitating fatigue experienced by some polio survivors may be related to aging of postencephalitic damaged neurons in the reticular activating system.[23] It is well-known not only that the polio virus damaged or killed anterior horn cells in the spinal cord but also that it affected a number of specific areas within the brain, including the reticular activating system. Dysfunction of this system with advancing age, especially when the system may have been partially damaged from the polioencephalitic infection a number of years previously, has been postulated as a cause for severe fatigue in some post-polio patients. This hypothesis is quite interesting, but much further investigation is needed before any definitive statements can be made. At the present time, it should be pointed out that, fortunately, rest and/or reduction in overall activity have been reported to ameliorate or abort the symptom.[10,23,45]

A few clinic reports provide information compatible with the concept that at least some of the complaints of fatigue expressed by post-polio patients are related to local muscular fatigue. For instance, Cosgrove and colleagues reported that the single most common complaint in patients seen in their post-polio clinic was that of decreasing endurance.[29] They reported that 153 out of 154 unstable post-polio patients (those complaining of progressive decline in muscular function) acknowledged progressive difficulty with endurance while performing their usual daily activities. Also, a recent survey reported that two-thirds of post-polio subjects complained of the increasing loss of strength during exercise and/or a heavy sensation of the muscles.[18] Both of these complaints are compatible with excessive local muscle fatigue.

The remainder of this chapter briefly reviews (1) proposed neurophysiologic and functional etiologies for decline in function in post-polio individuals, which may make it progressively more difficult for an individual to perform usual daily activities and possibly lead to problems with fatigue; (2) what is known about neuromuscular function and local muscle fatigue in polio survivors; (3) the effects of exercise in post-polio patients; and (4) some functional and clinical implications of this information, which may provide some useful guidelines, based upon physiological principles, regarding the treatment of post-polio individuals with fatigue-related problems.

PROPOSED NEUROPHYSIOLOGIC ETIOLOGIES FOR DECLINE IN NEUROMUSCULAR FUNCTION

A number of neurophysiologic etiologies have been proposed for late-onset deterioration in neuromuscular function in polio survivors,[52] and loss of strength over time can certainly lead to complaints related to poor endurance and greater fatigability. The latter concept is discussed in more detail later. These proposed etiologies include chronic or reactivated polio virus, scarring within the motor neurons leading to progressive dysfunction with aging, dysfunction due to excessive metabolic demand placed on the remaining motor neurons, loss of motor units with the normal aging process, and loss of muscle fibers within the enlarged reinnervated motor units.

REACTIVATED VIRUS, SCARRING, EXCESSIVE METABOLIC DEMAND

Chronic and/or reactivated poliovirus has been hypothesized in the past to be a cause for loss of function in polio survivors, but that theory has been essentially universally rejected.[42] It may certainly be the case, however, that surviving motor neurons are permanently scarred from the initial poliomyelitis infection, and, with the greater load that is placed on the enlarged surviving motor units, the motor units may not be able to keep pace with the metabolic demands of innervating all of their muscle fibers.[25,92] It has been shown both that the motor units in post-polio individuals have increased by up to sevenfold the normal size[37] and that such enlarged units may have difficulty in nourishing all of their muscle fibers within the surviving units. In this context, it is interesting to note that postmortem pathologic evaluation of eight patients, aged 36–61 years, who had had poliomyelitis and died of nonneurologic disease 9 months to 44 years after the acute poliomyelitis infection, revealed evidence of ongoing neuronal activity regardless of the presence or absence of new weakness in the individual before death.[76] These authors reported finding axonal spheroids only in individuals with new muscle weakness (i.e., patients with post-polio progressive muscle atrophy [PPMA]). And, as axonal spheroids have been reported to represent a defect in the movement of trophic materials from the neuron down the body of the axon[41] and are found predominantly in patients with motor neuron disease with recent neuronal deterioration,[24] it was suggested that PPMA might be the end of the spectrum of an ongoing neuronal reaction that slowly affects the ability of the surviving motor neurons to maintain the integrity of the distal nerve terminals.[76]

LOSS OF MOTOR UNITS

A decline in the number of anterior horn cells has been shown to be a part of the normal aging process. After the age of 60, the number of anterior horn cells has been shown to decline.[87] It is certainly most probable that a minor and unrecordable decline in the number of motor units occurs prior to the age of 60, but in the normal individual, the functional consequences of this may be unnoticeable. In the post-polio individual, however, with significant deficits already, the impact of this may be quite apparent. At an advanced age, this is most likely one of the major causes of recognized new weakness in post-polio individuals. The already enlarged motor units may have a limited capacity for reinnervation compared to what normally occurs in aging muscle.

LOSS OF MUSCLE FIBERS WITHIN THE MOTOR UNITS

To date, there is histologic,[25,43] immunohistochemical,[25] and electrophysiologic evidence[25,30,31,37,63,77,88,91,92] documenting the ongoing process of denervation and reinnervation of muscle fibers within the motor units even decades after acute poliomyelitis. Evidence of instability, however, has not been able to distinguish between stable post-polio patients and post-polio patients with complaints of new weakness.[25,30,37,63,77,92] Intuitively, the newly reinnervated muscle fibers may have a reduced capacity to function. This may be related to (1) dysfunctional, newly forming motor endplates that may have presynaptic and/or postsynaptic difficulties in providing the muscle fiber with the stimulus to contract, (2) reduced metabolic ability of the newly reinnervated muscle fibers to perform endurance activity, and/or (3) incomplete reinnervation. Any of these mechanisms may lead to progressive loss of strength or endurance; further investigation is required to document the specific mechanism(s).

PROPOSED FUNCTIONAL ETIOLOGIES FOR DECLINE IN NEUROMUSCULAR FUNCTION

A number of functional etiologies have also been proposed that may lead to an apparent loss of neuromuscular function.[11] These factors include progressive loss in strength and/or endurance from disuse or overuse, insidious weight gain, and chronic weakness of which the individual was perhaps unaware until post-polio syndrome became a well-known entity.

DISUSE WEAKNESS

It is well-known that disuse leads to a decrease in muscle strength and cardiorespiratory fitness. Müller demonstrated that young, healthy individuals can lose 20% of their strength with one week of immobilization.[67] Saltin and colleagues demonstrated that young healthy individuals can lose 25% of their cardiorespiratory fitness with three weeks of bed rest.[83]

There is indirect evidence to suggest that disuse may play a role in loss of neuromuscular function, at least in some post-polio individuals. Grimby and colleagues reported a low concentration of an aerobic enzyme, citrate synthase, in the quadriceps muscle of post-polio subjects, and this was believed to be compatible with a low level of activity among these individuals, as activity is known to increase the concentration of aerobic enzymes within the muscle.[43] Borg and Henriksson reported low concentrations of both citrate synthase and phosphofructokinase, a glycolytic enzyme, as well as a decrease in the capillary density in the tibialis anterior muscles of post-polio individuals.[21] It was believed that overall low muscle usage resulted in these findings and that low capillary density and decreased oxidative and glycolytic enzyme concentrations might be important factors in the development of muscle weakness, fatigue, and pain. A clinical report showed that the concentration of high-density lipoprotein cholesterol (HDL-C) was significantly reduced in post-polio men,[9] which was thought to be compatible with reduced activity in these individuals, as activity is known to increase HDL-C concentration. In another clinical report, 44% of patients seen in a post-polio clinic with complaints of post-polio syndrome acknowledged that their decline in function had begun at a time of hospitalization.[10] Although not proven, the disuse brought on by bed rest could have led to further loss in function, from which the patient could not fully recover. This may be an especially perplexing problem, as reactivation after immobilization may lead to overuse problems.

OVERUSE WEAKNESS

The concept of overuse is not new, although the mechanisms for it are not yet well understood. There are probably several different physiologic mechanisms responsible for overuse. These mechanisms may include both metabolic fatigue of the muscle and anatomic disruption of muscle fibers from overwork.

There are several anecdotal reports of overuse weakness in post-polio patients. In 1915, Lovett reported that activity led to deterioration rather than the expected usual improvement in strength in some polio survivors.[60] He noted that deterioration correlated with the activity of the individual; the greater the activity, the greater the deterioration in strength. Bennett and Knowlton cited five cases of post-polio patients' losing function with excessive activity, which those authors believed to be evidence of overuse weakness.[17,54]

Several reports in the literature indirectly implicate chronic muscle overuse in post-polio patients. In a study of energy expenditure and orthotics usage, Luna-Reyes and colleagues reported that the energy consumption of ambulation—as measured in kilocalories per kilogram of body weight per meter walked—by post-polio children with leg weakness was three times as great when a leg brace was not used.[61] In a kinesiologic study, Borg and colleagues reported that some polio survivors recruited their tibialis anterior muscle maximally or near maximally when walking, which could lead to overuse fatigue.[20] In another kinesiologic study, Perry and colleagues evaluated 34 unstable post-polio patients by using dynamic electromyography of several lower extremity muscle groups during ambulation. On the average, subjects had increased use of two muscle groups, which data further supported the concept of muscle overuse.[75] In another study, it was shown that patients who complained of progressive loss in strength were ones who had histories of a more widespread acute paralysis, but relatively greater functional recovery; were less disabled; and acknowledged higher levels of recent activity.[53] It is certainly possible, although unproven in these individuals, that the higher level of activity led to overuse problems and, subsequently, to their complaints of declining function. In a recent dynamometric study, it was reported that unstable post-polio subjects, compared to stable post-polio or control (nonpolio) subjects, had a deficit in recovery of muscle strength after fatiguing exercise.[5] It was concluded that the deficit in strength recovery was related to greater local muscle fatigue.[79]

Animal studies have demonstrated that anatomic disruption of the muscle fibers can occur from excessive use,[89] but there is no compelling evidence in the literature to indicate that this is the case in post-polio patients. Damage to muscle fibers can result in an elevation of the concentration of muscle enzymes in the blood, such as creatine kinase (CK). Two studies have reported that the mean concentration of CK was increased in unstable post-polio subjects;[71,90] however, the significance of this is unknown. In one of the studies, both unstable and stable post-polio patients were assessed.[71] The incidence of elevation of CK was not different between the stable and the unstable post-polio patients, and the elevation in CK concentration did not correlate with new or residual weakness.

WEIGHT GAIN

Weight gain, as a result of an increase in adipose tissue, is well-known to occur as individuals age. The insidious increase in weight will, of course, make it more difficult for the individual to perform many ADLs. Although the literature contains little information on weight gain in post-polio patients, there is good reason to believe that this is a significant problem for many such individuals (especially because of the difficulty that many post-polio individuals have in the performance of ADLs and because of a sedentary lifestyle, which may lead to an accumulation of adipose tissue). One clinical report indicated that 60% of the patients studied acknowledged recent weight gain.[10]

CHRONIC WEAKNESS

Years ago, Beasley demonstrated that post-polio patients with apparently "normal" strength as determined by manual muscle testing[64] had significant deficits when strength was determined quantitatively (Fig. 2).[16] The average post-polio patient with "normal" muscle strength as determined by manual muscle testing had a 50% deficit in strength when measured quantitatively. In fact, some of these patients with "normal" strength actually had up to an 80% deficit in muscle strength. Such a deficit may be compounded by the insidious effects of weight gain and the aging process. Recent studies, using quantitative methodology, have also confirmed that post-polio individuals are much weaker than the normal population.[5,35,36]

In a post-polio individual, the combination of disuse of some muscles and overuse of others, compounded by insidious weight gain and chronic weakness, can certainly contribute to progressive loss of functional capabilities, especially when the aging factor is also included. And these factors, in combination, can lead to further problems with fatigue.

EVIDENCE OF PROGRESSIVE LOSS OF STRENGTH

Although the development of late-onset weakness in polio survivors was first reported more than a century ago,[28,78] today there is little objective evidence in the literature to indicate that the rate of loss in strength is greater than that expected as a result of the aging process. In several investigations, the determination of progressive loss in strength was made

FIGURE 2. Manual muscle testing error of grading knee extension. (From Beasley WC: Quantitative clinical muscle testing: with emphasis upon estimating level of paresis relative to a standardized normal value. An exhibit presented at the Third International Congress of Physical Medicine Meeting. Washington, D.C., August 21–26, 1960.)

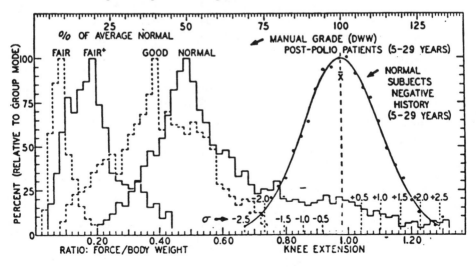

by patient report and not by longitudinal studies using valid and reliable measures. None of three reports in the referred literature that used valid and reliable measures for determination of strength in polio survivors found any loss in strength.[6,69,70] However, one of those studies assessed only six patients over a time span of 400 to 2,100 days,[70] another assessed the strength in 34 post-polio subjects over 1 year,[6] and the third assessed seven patients 3 years.[69] With few subjects in two of the studies and the short duration of the third, it is not surprising that none of the studies detected any significant loss in strength. A more recent study, however, over a 3-year follow-up period showed that both stable and unstable post-polio individuals had lost significant strength in the quadriceps femoris muscles but had not lost significant strength in the biceps humerus muscles.[8] The rate of loss of strength in the quadriceps, however, was no greater than that found in control (nonpolio) subjects. Thus, at this time it cannot be stated that the loss of strength is directly related to poliomyelitis and may instead be a reflection of the aging process. Obviously, further study is needed.

QUANTITATIVE ASSESSMENT OF STRENGTH, ENDURANCE, AND FATIGUE

MEASUREMENT BY DYNAMOMETRIC AND ELECTROMYOGRAPHIC TECHNIQUES

The function of the quadriceps femoris muscles was studied in 41 nonpolio (control), 34 unstable post-polio (those complaining of progressive decline in strength), and 16 stable post-polio (those not complaining of progressive decline in strength) subjects.[5,79,80] All subjects were healthy and were between the ages of 30 and 60 years at the onset of the study. All of the unstable post-polio subjects were complaining of progressive loss of muscle strength and/or endurance in general. In addition, most of the unstable post-polio subjects acknowledged that the quadriceps muscle evaluated in this study was losing strength and/or endurance; the stable post-polio subjects denied such symptoms. All of the post-polio subjects had greater than antigravity strength in the quadriceps on manual muscle testing.[64] The strength, endurance, work capacity, and ability to recover strength after exhausting activity were determined in the quadriceps muscles of all subjects. The quadriceps muscles also were studied electromyographically in order to look for evidence of old polio as well as evidence of new denervation in the post-polio subjects.

Those in the unstable group were significantly older than those in the stable group at the time of their original poliomyelitis illness (8.1 ± 6.2 vs. 4.7 ± 3.8 years, mean ± SD, respectively) and at the time of their maximal recovery following the acute polio illness (16.4 ± 8.1 vs. 9.7 ± 6.3 years, respectively). Although there was no difference between the two groups in the proportion of subjects hospitalized during their acute illness, the duration of hospitalization during the acute illness was significantly longer for those in the unstable than for those in the stable group (5.1 ± 4.4 vs. 1.2 ± 0.8 months, respectively). These findings demonstrate that the unstable subjects were older at the time of their acute illness, were hospitalized four times longer, and recovered more slowly than the stable subjects. The last two findings are certainly compatible with a more severe acute poliomyelitis illness in the unstable post-polio subjects, and they parallel the data of Halstead and Rossi.[45] Further evidence that unstable subjects had a more severe initial poliomyelitis illness was found by means of the electromyographic studies. Evidence of greater loss of motor neurons at the time of the acute poliomyelitis illness was found in the unstable post-polio group, but there was no difference between the two post-polio groups in evidence of new denervation.[5]

Strength and endurance testing revealed that the unstable post-polio group had significant deficits in neuromuscular function (Table 2). Muscle strength was found to be much less in the unstable group. On average, the unstable group had only approximately 50% of normal strength (i.e., the average strength of the control group), whereas the stable group had approximately 75% of normal strength. However, the isometric endurance time (the amount of time that subjects could contract the quadriceps muscle at 40% of maximum strength until they were no longer able to do so) was not significantly different among the three groups. On the other hand, the isometric "work capacity" (the amount of "work" the muscle performed during this endurance test) was significantly less in the unstable post-polio group than in the other two groups. The unstable post-polio group had only approximately 50% of normal work capacity, whereas the stable post-polio group had a work capacity similar to the controls'. Work capacity was found to be related to the strength of the muscle (Fig. 3). The analyses showed no difference among the three groups in work capacity when muscle strength was taken into consideration.

During the isometric endurance exercise to exhaustion, two electrophysiologic measures of local muscle fatigue were monitored (median frequency of the power spectrum and root mean squared amplitude of the electromyographic signal, from which the neuromuscular efficiency could be determined),[34,56,59,65] and at regular intervals throughout the test, subjects reported their rating of perceived exertion,[19] which indicated their perception of exertion in the muscle as a result of the exercise being per-

TABLE 2. Mean (±SD) Strength, Endurance Time, and Work Capacity of Unstable Post-Polio (Unstable), Stable Post-Polio (Stable), and Control Subjects

Variable	Unstable (n = 34)	Stable (n = 16)	Control (n = 41)
Knee extension Strength (Nm)	113 ± 75*	159 ± 87†	207 ± 61
Endurance time (sec)‡	102 ± 36	116 ± 52	119 ± 39
Work capacity (Nmsec)	5024 ± 3213[1]*	8221 ± 4140	9826 ± 4144

*Unstable significantly (p<0.05) less than Stable and Control.
†Stable significantly (p<0.05) less than Control.
‡No significant (p>0.05) difference among the three groups.

formed. No difference was found among the three groups in the electrophysiologic measures of local muscle fatigue.

Figure 4 depicts the change in the median frequency of the power spectrum of the surface recorded signal and the neuromuscular efficiency measured from the quadriceps muscle from the onset of the fatiguing contraction to the completion of the activity. Of significant clinical importance, the RPE did not differ among the three groups; that is, all subjects

FIGURE 3. Correlation of work capacity (in Nmsec) to isometric muscle strength (in nm) for unstable, stable, and control subjects. Correlation for each group is significant (p<.05). No significant (p>.05) difference among groups in slope of regression lines. (Adapted from Agre JC, Rodriquez AA: Neuromuscular function: Comparison of symptomatic and asymptomatic polio subjects to control subjects. Arch Phys Med Rehabil 71:545–551, 1990, with permission.)

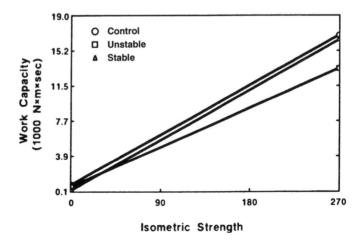

Isometric Strength

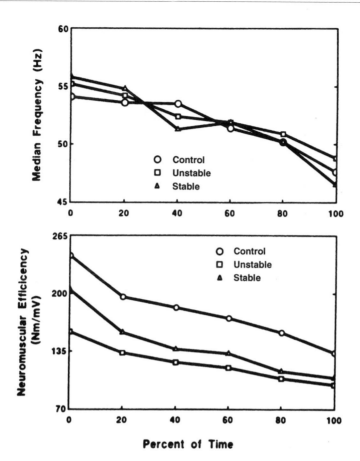

FIGURE 4. Mean change in neuromuscular efficiency (NME) and median frequency of the power spectrum (Fm) during the endurance test from onset (0%) to exhaustion (100%) in unstable post-polio, stable post-polio, and control subjects. No significant ($p > .05$) differences were found among groups for either variable. (Adapted from Rodriquez AA, Agre JC: Electrophysiologic study of the quadriceps muscles during fatiguing exercise and recovery: A comparison of symptomatic postpolios to asymptomatic postpolios and controls. Arch Phys Med Rehabil 72:993–997, 1991, with permission.)

could similarly perceive the extent of fatigue within the muscle throughout the exercise period, from the onset of the exercise all the way to the point of exhaustion (Fig. 5). In addition, the RPE and the electrophysiologic variables of local muscle fatigue were found to be related. As the subject reported that the perception of fatigue within the muscle was increasing, the electrophysiologic variables demonstrated that the muscle was indeed becoming more fatigued. Figure 6 provides an example of that finding in the unstable post-polio subjects.

Post-endurance testing revealed that the unstable post-polio subjects recovered strength significantly less readily than the control group,

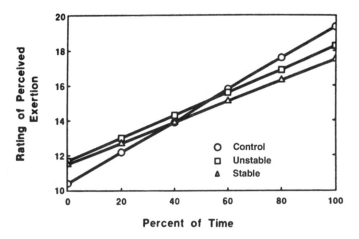

Percent of Time

FIGURE 5. A comparison of the mean change in rating of perceived exertion (RPE) during the endurance test from onset (0%) to exhaustion (100%). No significant ($p > .05$) difference among groups. (Adapted from Agre JC, Rodriquez AA: Neuromuscular function: Comparison of symptomatic and asymptomatic polio subjects to control subjects. Arch Phys Med Rehabil 71:545–551, 1990, with permission.)

whereas the stable post-polio group recovered strength similar to the control group (Fig 7). The deficit in strength recovery in the unstable group, however, did not appear to be due to lassitude or lack of volition, and it was consistent with greater local muscle fatigue in these subjects as there was no difference in the amplitude of the relative root mean squared electromyographic amplitude during this recovery testing (Fig. 8). The sub-

FIGURE 6. Interaction between rating of perceived exertion (RPE) and median frequency of the power spectrum (Fm) in the unstable post-polio group. Interaction is statistically significant ($p < .05$). (From Rodriquez AA, Agre JC: Physiologic parameters and perceived exertion with local muscle fatigue in postpolio subjects. Arch Phys Med Rehabil 72:305–308, 1991, with permission.)

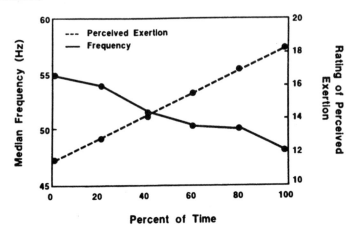

Percent of Time

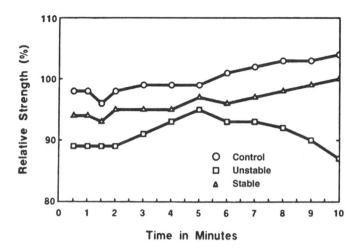

FIGURE 7. A comparison of recovery of mean relative isometric strength from 30 seconds to 10 minutes after exhaustion. Unstable subjects differed significantly ($p<.05$) from control subjects. Stable subjects and controls did not significantly ($p>.05$) differ. (Adapted from Agre JC, Rodriquez AA: Neuromuscular function: Comparison of symptomatic and asymptomatic polio subjects to control subjects. Arch Phys Med Rehabil 71:545–551, 1990, with permission.)

FIGURE 8. Mean change in root mean squared electromyogram (RMS-EMG) amplitude after exhaustion in unstable post-polio, stable post-polio, and control subjects. Measurements were made in intervals from 30 seconds to 10 minutes post exhaustion. No significant ($p>.05$) difference was found among the three groups. (Adapted from Rodriquez AA, Agre JC: Electrophysiologic study of the quadriceps muscles during fatiguing exercise and recovery: A comparison of symptomatic postpolios to asymptomatic postpolios and controls. Arch Phys Med Rehabil 72:993–997, 1991, with permission.)

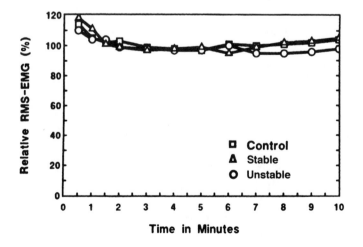

jective time to completely recover from this fatiguing exercise was also significantly longer in the unstable post-polio group. In the stable post-polio and the control (nonpolio) groups, recovery usually occurred within one day; in the unstable post-polio group, recovery usually did not occur until two to three days after the activity.[7]

TABLE 3. Features from the Literature Delineating Similarities and Differences Between Stable and Unstable Post-polio Individuals

Similarities	Reference(s)
1. Evidence of denervation/reinnervation of muscle fibers in motor units	Wiechers & Hubbel, 1981[92] Cruz Martinez et al, 1984[30] Cashman et al, 1987[25] Einarsson et al, 1990[37] Ravits et al, 1990[77] Maselli et al, 1992[63]
2. Incidence of elevated serum creatine kinase	Nelson, 1990[71]
3. Muscular endurance (while performing exercise at a similar relative level of exertion)	Agre & Rodriquez, 1990[5]
4. Electrophysiologic evidence of local muscle fatigue (while performing exercise at a similar relative level of exertion)	Rodriquez & Agre, 1991[79]
5. Rating of perceived exertion (while performing exercise at a similar relative level of exertion)	Agre & Rodriquez, 1991[5]
6. Rate of loss in strength over time?	Agre et al, 1992[8]

Differences	Reference(s)
1. Evidence of more widespread initial poliomyelitis illness in unstable post-polio individuals	Klingman et al, 1988[53] Halstead & Rossi, 1985[45]
2. Unstable post-polio individuals had their acute illness at an older age	Halstead & Rossi, 1985[45] Agre & Rodriquez, 1990[5]
3. Unstable post-polio individuals hospitalized longer at the time of their acute polio illness	Halstead & Rossi, 1985[45] Agre & Rodriquez, 1990[5]
4. Unstable post-polio individuals acknowledge higher level of recent activity	Klingman et al, 1988[53]
5. Unstable post-polio individuals have weaker muscles	Agre & Rodriquez, 1990[5]
6. Unstable post-polio individuals have reduced capacity for muscular work	Agre & Rodriquez, 1990[5]
7. Unstable post-polio individuals have a deficit in strength recovery after fatiguing exercise	Agre & Rodriquez, 1990[5] Agre et al, 1991[7]

MEASUREMENT OF ^{31}P MAGNETIC RESONANCE SPECTROSCOPY DURING LOW- AND HIGH-INTENSITY HANDGRIP EXERCISE

One study utilized ^{31}P magnetic resonance spectroscopy to determine whether there was a difference at rest and after low- or high-intensity handgrip exercise in the concentration of high-energy phosphates or pH in the forearm muscles of post-polio and control subjects.[85] This technique has been reported to show metabolic abnormalities in patients with muscle denervation[95] and with chronic fatigue.[86] Seventeen post-polio and 28 control subjects were studied. Although the post-polio group's response to exercise was highly variable, no significant differences were found between the groups at rest or after exercise. The authors concluded that their data suggested that the whole-body fatigue experienced by polio survivors was not related to any systemic metabolic abnormality.

In both of the aforementioned studies, no differences were found comparing the post-polio to the control muscle during the fatiguing process in any measured variable, including psychophysiologic (the RPE), electrophysiologic (median frequency of the power spectrum and neuromuscular efficiency), and magnetic resonance spectroscopic measurements. The later measurements are utilized to indirectly assess the metabolic processes during fatiguing muscular activity and the former is the subjective evaluation by the subject for the level of exertion within the exercising muscle. It thus appears that the post-polio muscle is reasonably well adapted and compensated from a physiologic standpoint. Nonetheless, in the one study that investigated recovery of strength after exhausting activity, the post-polio muscle has been shown to recover strength much less readily than the normal muscle either while the measurements are made in the laboratory[5,79] or as determined subjectively by the subjects thereafter.[7] The precise reason for this is as yet unknown, but from the available data, it appears to be peripheral rather than central in nature.

BENEFICIAL EFFECT OF PACING ON MUSCLE FUNCTION

Although it was found that unstable post-polio subjects had significantly less strength and less work capacity and that they recovered strength less readily than control subjects, they could perceive fatigue in the muscle as well as the control subjects could.[5] This seems to indicate that post-polio subjects could avoid excessive local muscle fatigue by pacing their activities (i.e., by interspersing rest breaks into their scheduled activities).

A study was performed to determine whether pacing (interspersion of rest breaks into activity) would allow unstable post-polio subjects both to perform similar or increased work with less local muscle fatigue and to increase their ability to recover strength after activity than when these same subjects worked constantly until exhaustion was reached.[4]

Seven unstable post-polio subjects were tested on three separate days with at least one week between tests. On the first test day, the strength and endurance exercise and recovery testing were performed as described previously. On the second test day, subjects performed the same amount of isometric work at the same relative level of intensity as they had on the first test day, but the exercise was divided into quartiles by 2-minute rest breaks. On the third test day, subjects performed 20-second intervals of isometric exercise at the same relative intensity, with 2-minute rest breaks between exercise intervals. Exercise continued until either perceived exertion was rated as greater than "very hard" or 18 intervals of isometric work had been performed.

At the onset of exercise for each of the three test paradigms there was no significant difference in the variables related to local muscle fatigue (electromyographic or RPE). However, at the completion of the exercise, both variables demonstrated significantly greater local muscle fatigue in the constant exercise paradigm compared to either the quartile or interval exercise paradigms (Fig. 9). In addition, the relative recovery of strength

FIGURE 9. Comparison of constant isometric exercise to quartile and interval isometric exercise with regard to EMG amplitude, median frequency (Fm), and rating of perceived exertion (RPE) in seven unstable post-polio subjects at onset and completion of each activity. The completion value for each variable is significantly ($p<.05$) different, comparing the constant exercise to either quartile exercise or interval exercise. (Adapted from Agre JC, Rodriquez AA: Intermittent isometric activity: Its effect on muscle fatigue in postpolio subjects. Arch Phys Med Rehabil 72:971–975, 1991, with permission.)

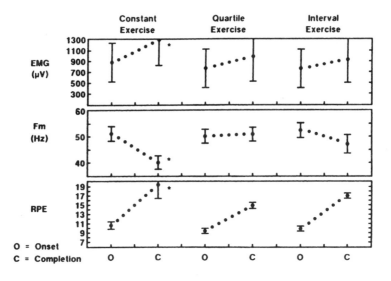

was significantly greater after quartile and interval exercise than after constant exercise. Also of note, the amount of isometric work performed during the interval exercise paradigm was significantly greater (237% on average) than during constant exercise. All of these findings indicate that pacing can result in significant reduction in local muscle fatigue even when similar or greater amounts of work are performed by unstable post-polio subjects.

EFFECT OF EXERCISE IN POST-POLIO PATIENTS

MUSCLE-STRENGTHENING EXERCISES

Several early studies have indicated that strengthening programs initiated weeks to a few years after the acute poliomyelitis illness were beneficial.[33,44,58,68,82] However, a number of case reports have reported that vigorous exercise or activity in that time period was detrimental.[17,50,54,66]

In a review article by Herbison and colleagues on exercise therapies in patients with peripheral neuropathies, it was concluded that brief isometric or isotonic contractions might be of greater benefit for muscle strength than a program of habitual exhausting exercise, because overwork might damage the partially denervated muscle.[49]

The results of studies conducted on muscle-strengthening exercise in the post-polio population are briefly reviewed below.

Feldman and Soskolne reported the effect of at least 24 weeks of nonfatiguing exercise on 32 muscle groups in six post-polio patients.[38] They reported that 14 muscles improved strength, 17 muscles maintained strength, and one muscle had decreased strength. Unfortunately, neither the specifics of the exercise program nor the results were delineated.

Einarsson and Grimby reported the effect of a standardized, 6-week, thrice-weekly, isokinetic and isometric strengthening exercise program on the quadriceps muscles of 12 post-polio subjects with grade 3+ or greater muscle strength on manual muscle testing.[35,36] Isokinetic and isometric strength increased significantly; citrate synthase concentration also increased, but not significantly. There was no evidence of damage to the muscle as a result of the exercise program as no changes were seen in histopathologic findings on muscle biopsies taken after training compared to before training.

Fillyaw and colleagues reported the effect of long-term nonfatiguing resistance exercise in 17 post-polio patients.[39] Maximum torque was reported to increase in the exercised muscles compared to the control muscles, in which no change in strength was found. Fillyaw and associates concluded that individuals with post-polio syndrome can increase muscle strength by doing nonfatiguing resistance exercise, but that they should undergo quantitative testing of muscle strength a minimum of every 3 months to guard against overwork weakness.

Agre and colleagues recently reported the effect of a closely supervised, 12-week, nonfatiguing quadriceps muscle–strengthening program in subjects with at least grade 3+ muscle strength on manual muscle testing.[3] Every other day, subjects performed 6–10 knee extension exercises with sandbag weights attached to the ankle, holding the weight for 5 seconds at full extension and then resting for 25 seconds before the next repetition. The weight was increased whenever the subject could perform 10 repetitions without reaching an RPE[19] of "very hard" in the muscle. After the 12 weeks of exercise, the average amount of weight a subject could lift had increased over 60%. No subject experienced problems with the exercise program and no change was found either in the concentration of serum CK or in the amount of jitter or blocking on electromyographic testing after the exercise program compared to beforehand. It was concluded that a carefully monitored and supervised exercise program could safely increase strength in post-polio individuals with at least grade 3+ strength.

CARDIORESPIRATORY AND GENERAL EXERCISE

From a cardiorespiratory standpoint, post-polio patients are known to be deconditioned. Owen and Jones reported that the aerobic power of the typical post-polio patient was similar to that of patients with recent myocardial infarction.[72] The average maximal metabolic capacity of these patients was only 5.6 metabolic equivalents (one metabolic equivalent is the energy expenditure of a subject at complete rest). Jones and colleagues reported responses to a 16-week, thrice-weekly, aerobic exercise program.[51] Sixteen subjects exercised on bicycle ergometers at an intensity of 70% of maximum heart rate. To avoid problems of muscle fatigue, exercise was performed in bouts of 2–5 minutes, with 1-minute rest breaks, and patients were instructed to exercise for 15–30 minutes per session. Training had to be started at somewhat lower intensity during the first weeks of the study and then could be slowly increased. Compared to 21 control post-polio subjects, who had no change in fitness, the exercise subjects increased work capacity by 18% and aerobic power by 15% and had no untoward responses to the exercise program. Subjectively, the exercise subjects noted a decrease in fatigue during their daily activities and a feeling of increased strength in the lower extremity muscles. It was concluded that post-polio patients could safely increase their aerobic fitness in a manner similar to that of healthy nonpolio adults.

Grimby and Einarsson reported the effect of a 6-month, twice-weekly exercise program in 12 post-polio subjects.[42] All subjects had had polio 28–44 years before the study and could walk, but one used a cane. All had significantly reduced strength in several muscle groups in their lower extremities. After a 5-minute warm-up, both walking and biking at submaximal levels were performed for 5–10 minutes. Thereafter, mobility and stretching exercises were performed and several different strengthening exercises were performed for individual muscle groups using body weight as resistance. The subjects were also advised about home programs and daily activities.

A bicycle ergometer showed that the exercise program had resulted in an improvement in peak exercise performance and that the heart rate at a submaximal workload was reduced. Muscle strength was found to increase in the elbow extensors and hip abductors, but not significantly in the knee extensors. Muscle fiber area and concentration of citrate synthase of the quadriceps did not significantly increase in the group, but some subjects showed an increase in knee extension strength, and their muscle fiber areas did increase. Evidence of overwork, however, was found in one subject, who had an unusually high proportion of type II muscle fibers; this is quite unexpected in post-polio patients. Objective measurements showed reduced strength and endurance during the training program, which also corresponded with subjective feelings of marked fatigue during and after the training sessions. The training continued due to the high motivation of the subject, who fully understood the risk attendant to participation. During the subsequent half year, with reduced level of activity, the subject's muscle strength returned toward pretraining values, with decrease in fatigue. It was concluded that an exercise program that combined endurance training, stretching, and submaximal strengthening exercises can be conducted in post-polio subjects with positive effects but that the cardiorespiratory condition effects in the program seemed to predominate. One subject had deleterious effects from the program, which resolved after the program by means of reduction in level of activity. This subject had experienced increased fatigue during the program. Thus, if a subject does not note a subjective increase in fatigue, such a program appears to be positive.

Dean and Ross reported the effect of a modified aerobic training program on movement energetics in post-polio individuals.[32] Their modified aerobic training program consisted of three training sessions per week for 6 weeks. Subjects walked on a treadmill for 20–40 minutes per session at a speed and grade that were comfortable for the subject (perceived exertion did not exceed "somewhat heavy," and pain was maintained at near 0

TABLE 4. Therapeutic Recommendations for Post-Polio Individuals to Better Control Their Symptoms of Fatigue

1. Weight loss, when appropriate
2. Protection of weakened muscles from overuse by use of appropriate adaptive equipment
3. Reduction of overall level of activity
4. Avoidance of excessive fatigue
5. Appropriate gentle exercise under supervision when disuse is suspected

and was never permitted to exceed "light"). Compared to the control group of 13 subjects, at the end of the study, the experimental group of seven subjects had greater movement economy (reduction in energy cost of walking) and walking duration. No change, however, was found in subjects' cardiorespiratory conditioning. It was concluded that a modified aerobic training program may have a role in enhancing endurance and reducing fatigue during ADL in post-polio individuals by improving their efficiency of movement.

FUNCTIONAL IMPLICATIONS

In this review, it has been shown that unstable post-polio subjects had a history of a more severe poliomyelitis illness that was corroborated electromyographically.[5] The unstable post-polio group was also much weaker than the stable post-polio group and, because of this, had a greatly reduced capacity to perform isometric work. However, endurance time was the same in the unstable post-polio, stable post-polio, and control (nonpolio) subjects when isometric work was performed at the same relative level of effort in all subjects.

It should be pointed out that post-polio subjects with significant weakness do not perform daily activities at the same *relative* level of effort as do other individuals, because the post-polio muscle may have to work at much closer to maximal strength in order to perform activities that nonpolio subjects can easily perform at a much lower relative level of effort. Furthermore, high-intensity effort is known to rapidly fatigue the muscle, with endurance time being less with greater relative exertion.[81] For instance, if a subject performs an isometric activity at 20% of maximal effort, endurance time has been shown to be approximately 10 minutes; at 40% of maximal effort, endurance time is approximately 2 minutes (Fig. 10).[81] Thus, an individual with half the strength of another subject (the average unstable post-polio subject in the previously cited studies) would have to work at twice the *relative effort* to perform the same *absolute* work as the stronger subject and have a significantly diminished endurance capacity.

It has also been shown that post-polio subjects do lose muscle strength in the quadriceps femoris muscles, although current research does not indicate that the rate of loss is any greater than that found among nonpolio control subjects of similar age. It should be pointed out, however, that the loss of strength in the post-polio individual may have a much greater impact on that individual than on other individuals. The post-polio individual must always perform an activity at a much higher relative level of effort, due to the muscle weakness. That is to say, the weak individual is

FIGURE 10. Endurance and intensity of work. Static work: tension at fractions of maximal strength. (From Simonson E: Physiology of Work Capacity and Fatigue. Springfield, IL, Charles C Thomas, 1971, pp 440–458. Redrawn from Rohmert W: Ermittlung von Erholungspausen für statische Arbeit des Menschen. Int Z Angew Physiol 18:1`23–164, 1960, with permission.)

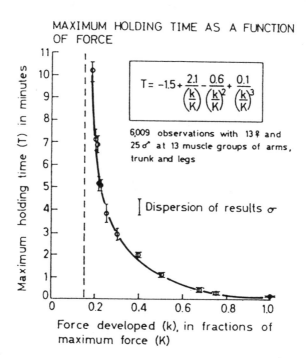

MAXIMUM HOLDING TIME AS A FUNCTION OF FORCE

$$T = -1.5 + \frac{2.1}{\left(\frac{k}{K}\right)} - \frac{0.6}{\left(\frac{k}{K}\right)^2} + \frac{0.1}{\left(\frac{k}{K}\right)^3}$$

6,009 observations with 13 ♀ and 25 ♂ at 13 muscle groups of arms, trunk and legs

∫ Dispersion of results σ

Maximum holding time (T) in minutes

Force developed (k), in fractions of maximum force (K)

always functioning at levels close to threshold. A "minor" loss of strength in such an individual may make it difficult, if not impossible, to continue to perform some daily activities, because the level of strength may drop below the threshold for ability to perform the activity.

Recent preliminary research data add further substantiation to the speculated relationship between muscle weakness and problems with fatigue. A study of 78 post-polio patients was performed to determine whether reduced muscle strength was related to fatigue as well as to post-polio syndrome (as defined by Halstead and Rossi),[46] difficulties with walking, and/or difficulties with stair climbing.[1,2] Strength of the quadriceps was assessed quantitatively initially and 4 years later. At the time of the second assessment, a questionnaire was completed regarding new symptomatology. It was found that subjects with complaints of new fatigue, of difficulty with walking or stair climbing, and of post-polio syndrome were significantly weaker at the time of the initial measurement as well as at the time of the final measurement compared to the other subjects. Although strength was found to significantly decline during the 4-year interval in the total group (by about 2% per year), the rate of loss was no different—comparing the group with the complaints—compared to the rate among the group without the complaints. It thus appears that post-polio individuals with complaints of fatigue are much weaker than those without complaints of fatigue.

In addition, research has shown both that unstable post-polio individuals have greater difficulty in recovering strength after an exhausting activity and that the subjective time to recover is two to three times as long as that among stable post-polio or control subjects.[5,7] Perhaps the combination of reduced strength and work capacity and the deficit in strength recovery due to excessive local muscle fatigue may be factors related to the unstable post-polio subject's complaints of fatigue and of progressive decline in neuromuscular function. In all events, the deficit in strength recovery certainly indicates that unstable post-polio subjects should avoid excessive local muscle fatigue.

CLINICAL IMPLICATIONS

It is of great clinical significance that the RPE was found to be similar in unstable post-polio, stable post-polio, and control subjects during an isometric endurance test.[5] This finding demonstrates that unstable post-polio subjects do have the ability to perceive muscular fatigue and can stop their activity prior to exhaustion. This perception may be used by the post-polio individual for pacing of activity to avoid excessive local muscle fatigue. And, as was described earlier, unstable post-polio subjects been shown to perform similar or greater exercise with less evidence of local muscle fatigue by pacing their activity.[4]

We highly recommend that post-polio individuals pace their daily activities to avoid excessive local muscle fatigue. Anecdotally, in the clinical setting, post-polio individuals acknowledge that pacing helps reduce pain[10,94] and fatigue.[10,73,94]

A recent study has reported the effect of compliance (the degree to which post-polio patients complied with clinically recommended interventions such as use of orthotics, lifestyle changes, weight loss, decrease in work hours, and aerobic exercise as appropriate for the patient's situation) on a number of factors, including fatigue.[74] Patients were divided into three groups based on the degree to which they complied with clinical recommendations: compliers ($n = 30$), partial compliers ($n = 32$), and noncompliers ($n = 15$). At the end of the follow-up period (an average of 2 years), 100% of compliers noted improvement or resolution of their complaint of fatigue; 68% of partial compliers reported improvement in fatigue, and only 3% an increase in fatigue; 0% of noncompliers reported improvement or resolution of fatigue; and 36% reported an increase in fatigue. It was concluded that compliance with recommendations significantly reduced symptomatology in post-polio patients, including the complaint of fatigue.

The recent exercise studies have shown that post-polio patients can benefit from strengthening as well as cardiovascular and general conditioning exercises, but the information should be interpreted with some caution. In all of the studies, the subjects were carefully monitored and the program was designed to be nonfatiguing in nature. As was pointed out by Grimby and Einarsson, even with such a program, exercise in these individuals can lead to overwork and further dysfunction that improves only with rest, rather than exercise.[42] At this time, one may conclude that anytime a post-polio individual begins an exercise program, that program should be carefully structured and monitored so that the individual does not develop further problems related to the exercise program.

CONCLUSIONS

Fatigue is a complex phenomenon and perhaps a complex of numerous phenomena. At this time, it is not well understood, but most certainly everyone experiences fatigue from time to time. In the post-polio population, however, fatigue is a very prevalent complaint, which appears to interfere with ability to function. The cause(s) for excessive fatigue in this population is (are) not precisely known at the present time but may be related to central as well as peripheral factors. It is known that unstable post-polio individuals, compared to stable post-polio and control (nonpolio) individuals, have measurable deficits in muscle strength, work capacity, and ability to recover strength after exhausting activity. It has also been shown that post-polio individuals do have a measurable loss of strength over time, but present research data show that it is at no greater a rate than that found in the nonpolio population. However, further loss of strength in an individual already significantly compromised may lead to greater difficulty in performing daily activities and with more fatigue related to those activities, as it is well-known that the closer one works to maximal functional capacity, the more quickly one fatigues.

A number of recommendations as follows may help the post-polio individual to better control symptoms of fatigue:

(1) Weight loss should be achieved in cases where adipose tissue has accumulated.

(2) Weakened muscles should be protected from overuse by appropriate adaptive equipment (use of orthotics, canes, wheelchairs, etc.). For instance, the use of simple pieces of adaptive equipment is known to significantly reduce the energy expenditure required for ambulation.

(3) The overall level of activity should be reduced; prioritize activities; less essential activities eliminated when need be; the day planned to more efficiently complete the essential daily activities; and intervals of activity interspersed with intervals of rest.

(4) Excessive fatigue should be avoided, as it has been shown that unstable post-polio individuals do not recover from exhausting activity as do others, and this problem appears to be related to excessive local muscle fatigue. It has been shown that it may take days for the unstable post-polio individual to fully recover from exhausting activity.

(5) When disuse is a part of the problem, appropriate gentle exercises such as stretching, strengthening, and cardiorespiratory fitness training may be quite helpful. The performance of such exercises should also be carried out via intervals of exercise interspersed with intervals of rest to avoid excessive fatigue, and the program should be carefully designed for the individual and carefully monitored.

REFERENCES

1. Agre JC, Grimby G, Einarsson G, et al: Relationship between muscle strength and complaints of new fatigue, new muscle weakness, or new muscle pain in postpolio survivors [abstract]. Arch Phys Med Rehabil 74:1261, 1993.

2. Agre JC, Grimby G, Einarsson G, et al: A comparison between postpolio individuals living in Sweden and the United States [abstract]. Arch Phys Med Rehabil 74:1261, 1993.

3. Agre JC, Harmon RL, Curt JT, et al: Nonfatiguing muscle strengthening exercise can safely increase strength in postpolio patients [abstract]. Med Sci Sports Exerc 25 (suppl):S134, 1993.

4. Agre JC, Rodriquez AA: Intermittent isometric activity: Its effect on muscle fatigue in postpolio subjects. Arch Phys Med Rehabil 72:971–975, 1991.

5. Agre JC, Rodriquez AA: Neuromuscular function: Comparison of symptomatic and asymptomatic polio subjects to control subjects. Arch Phys Med Rehabil 71:545–551, 1990.

6. Agre JC, Rodriquez AA: Neuromuscular function in polio survivors at one-year follow-up. Arch Phys Med Rehabil 72:7–10, 1991.

7. Agre JC, Rodriquez AA, Franke TM, Knudtson ER: Recovery time after exhausting muscular exercise in postpolio and control subjects [abstract]. Arch Phys Med Rehabil 72:778, 1991.

8. Agre JC, Rodriquez AA, Franke TM, et al: A three-year follow-up study of neuromuscular function in postpolio subjects [abstract]. Med Sci Sports Exerc 24(suppl):S73, 1992.

9. Agre JC, Rodriquez AA, Sperling KB: Plasma lipid and liproprotein concentrations in symptomatic postpolio patients. Arch Phys Med Rehabil 71:393–394, 1990.

10. Agre JC, Rodriquez AA, Sperling KB: Symptoms and clinical impressions of patients seen in a postpolio clinic. Arch Phys Med Rehabil 70:367–370, 1989.

11. Agre JC, Rodriquez AA, Tafel JA: Late effects of polio: Critical review of the literature on neuromuscular function. Arch Phys Med Rehabil 72:923–931, 1991.

12. American Heritage Dictionary, 2nd college ed. Boston, Houghton Mifflin Company, 1982, p 492.

13. Asmussen E: Muscle fatigue. Med Sci Sports Exerc 11:313–321, 1979.

14. Åstrand P-O, Rodahl K: Textbook of Work Physiology: Physiological Bases of Exercise. New York, McGraw-Hill, 1977.

15. Basmajian JV: Muscular tone, fatigue and neural influences. In Basmajian JV: Muscles Alive: Their Functions Revealed by Electromyography, 4th ed. Baltimore, Williams & Wilkins, 1978, pp 79–114.

16. Beasley WC: Quantitative muscle testing: Principles and applications for research and clinical services. Arch Phys Med Rehabil 42:398–425, 1961.

17. Bennett RL, Knowlton GC: Overwork weakness in partially denervated skeletal muscle. Clin Orthop 12:22–29, 1958.

18. Berlly MH, Strauser WW, Hall KM: Fatigue in postpolio syndrome. Arch Phys Med Rehabil 72:115–118, 1991.

19. Borg GAV: Perceived exertion: A note on "history" and methods. Med Sci Sports Exerc 5:90–93, 1973.

20. Borg K, Borg J, Edstrom L, Grimby L: Effects of excessive use of remaining muscle fibers in prior polio and LV lesion. Muscle Nerve 11:1219–1230, 1988.

21. Borg K, Henriksson J: Prior poliomyelitis-reduced capillary supply and metabolic enzyme content in hypertrophic slow-twitch (type I) muscle fibers. J Neurol Neurosurg Psychiatry 54:236–240, 1991.

22. Bruno RL, Frick NM: The psychology of polio as prelude to post-polio sequelae: Behavior modification and psychotherapy. Orthopedics 14:1185–1193, 1991.

23. Bruno RL, Frick NM, Cohen J: Polioencephalitis and the etiology of post-polio sequelae. Orthopedics 14:1269–1276, 1991.

24. Carpenter S: Proximal axonal enlargement in motor neuron disease. Neurology 18:842–851, 1968.

25. Cashman NR, Maselli R, Wollmann RL, et al: Late denervation in patients with antecedent paralytic poliomyelitis. N Engl J Med 317:7–12, 1987.

26. Codd MB, Mulder DW, Kurland LT, et al: Poliomyelitis in Rochester, Minnesota, 1935–1955: Epidemiology and long-term sequelae: A preliminary report. In Halstead LS, Wiechers DO, eds: Late Effects of Poliomyelitis. Miami, Symposia Foundation, 1985, pp. 121–134.

27. Conrady LJ, Wish JR, Agre JC, et al: Psychologic characteristics of polio survivors: A preliminary report. Arch Phys Med Rehabil 70:458–463, 1989.

28. Lepine C: Sur un cas de paralysie générale spinale antérieure subaigue, suivi d'autopsie. Gaz Med Fr (Paris) 4:127–129, 1875.

29. Cosgrove JL, Alexander MA, Kitts EL, et al: Late effects of poliomyelitis. Arch Phys Med Rehabil 68:4–7, 1987.

30. Cruz Martinez MA, Ferrer MT, Perez Conde MC: Electrophysiological features in patients with non-progressive and late progressive weakness after paralytic poliomyelitis: Electromyogram and single fiber electromyography study. Electromyogr Clin Neurophys 24:469–479, 1984.

31. Dalakas MB, Elder G, Hallat M, et al: A long-term follow-up study of patients with post-poliomyelitis neuromuscular symptoms. N Engl J Med 314:959–963, 1986.

32. Dean E, Ross J: Effect of modified aerobic training on movement energetics in polio survivors. Orthopedics 14:1243–1246, 1991.

33. DeLorme TL, Schwab RS, Watkins AL: The response of the quadriceps femoris to progressive resistance exercises in polio myelitic patients. J Bone Joint Surg (Am) 30:834–847, 1948.

34. DeLuca CJ: Myoelectric manifestations of localized muscular fatigue in humans. Crit Rev Biomed Eng 11:251–279, 1985.

35. Einarsson G: Muscle conditioning in late poliomyelitis. Arch Phys Med Rehabil 72:11–14, 1991.

36. Einarsson G, Grimby G: Strengthening exercise program in post-polio subjects. In Halstead LS, Wiechers DO (eds): Research and Clinical Aspects of the Late Effects of Poliomyelitis. Birth Defects 23(4):275–283, 1987.

37. Einarsson G, Grimby G, Stålberg E: Electromyographic and morphological functional compensation in late poliomyelitis. Muscle Nerve 13:165–171, 1990.

38. Feldman RM, Soskolne CL: The use of nonfatiguing strengthening exercises in post-polio syndrome. In Halstead LS, Wiechers DO (eds): Research and Clinical Aspects of the Late Effects of Poliomyelitis. Birth Defects 23(4):335–341, 1987.

39. Fillyaw MJ, Badger GJ, Goodwin GD, et al: The effects of long-term non-fatiguing resistance exercise in subjects with post-polio syndrome. Orthopedics 14:1253–1256, 1991.

40. Frick NM: Post-polio sequelae and psychology of second disability. Orthopedics 8:851–853, 1985.

41. Griffin JW, Price DL: Proximal axonopathies induced by toxic chemicals. In Spencer PS, Schaumburg HH (eds): Experimental and Clinical Neurotoxicology. Baltimore, Williams & Wilkins, 1980, pp 161–178.

42. Grimby G, Einarsson G: Post-polio management. CRC Crit Rev Phys Med Rehabil 2:189–200, 1991.

43. Grimby G, Einarsson G, Hedberg M, Aniansson A: Muscle adaptive changes in post-polio subjects. Scand J Rehabil Med 21:19–26, 1989.

44. Gurewitsch AD: Intensive graduated exercises in early infantile paralysis. Arch Phys Med 31:213–218, 1950.

45. Halstead LS, Rossi CD: New problems in old polio patients: Results of a survey of 539 polio survivors. Orthopedics 8:845–850, 1985.

46. Halstead LS, Rossi CD: Postpolio syndrome: Clinical experience with 132 consecutive outpatients. In Halstead LS, Wiechers DO (eds): Research and Clinical Aspects of the Late Effects of Poliomyelitis. Birth Defects 23(4):13–26, 1987.

47. Halstead LS, Wiechers DO (eds): Late Effects of Poliomyelitis. Miami, Symposia Foundation, 1985.

48. Halstead LS, Wiechers DO (eds): Research and Clinical Aspects of the Late Effects of Poliomyelitis. Birth Defects 23(4):1–363, 1987.

49. Herbison GJ, Jaweed MM, Ditunno JF Jr: Exercise therapies in peripheral neuropathies. Arch Phys Med Rehabil 64:201–205, 1983.

50. Hyman G: Poliomyelitis. Lancet 1:852, 1953.

51. Jones DR, Speier J, Canine K, et al: Cardiorespiratory responses to aerobic training by patients with postpoliomyelitis sequelae. JAMA 261:3255–3258, 1989.

52. Jubelt B, Cashman NR: Neurological manifestations of the post-polio syndrome. CRC Crit Rev Clin Neurobiol 3:199–220, 1987.

53. Klingman J, Chui H, Corgiat M, Perry J: Functional recovery: A major risk factor for development of postpoliomyelitis muscular atrophy. Arch Neurol 45:645–647, 1988.

54. Knowlton GC, Bennett RL: Overwork. Arch Phys Med Rehabil 38:18–20, 1957.

55. Kohl SJ: Emotional responses to the late effects of poliomyelitis. In Halstead LS, Wiechers DO (eds): Research and Clinical Aspects of the Late Effects of Poliomyelitis. Birth Defects 23(4):137–145, 1987.

56. Komi PV, Tesch P: EMG frequency spectrum during dynamic contractions in man. Eur J Appl Physiol 42:41–50, 1979.

57. Lange DJ, Smith T, Lovelace RE: Postpolio muscular atrophy: Diagnostic utility of macroelectromyography. Arch Neurol 46:502–506, 1989.

58. Lenman JAR: A clinical and experimental study of the effects of exercise on motor weakness in neurological disease. J Neurol Neurosurg Psychiatry 22:182–194, 1959.

59. Lindstrom L, Magnusson R, Peterson I: Muscular fatigue and action potential conduction velocity changes studied with frequency analysis of EMG signals. Electromyography 4:341–356, 1970.

60. Lovett RW: The treatment of infantile paralysis: Preliminary report, based on a study of the Vermont epidemic of 1914. JAMA 64:2118–2123, 1915.

61. Luna-Reyes OB, Reyes TM, So MLFY, et al: Energy cost of ambulation in healthy and disabled Filipino children. Arch Phys Med Rehabil 69:946–949, 1988.

62. MacLaren DPM, Gibson H, Parry-Billings M, Edwards RHT: A review of metabolic and physiological factors in fatigue. Sport Sci Rev 17:29–66, 1989.

63. Maselli RA, Cashman NR, Wollman RL, et al: Neuromuscular transmission as a function of motor unit size in patients with prior poliomyelitis. Muscle Nerve 15:648–655, 1992.

64. Medical Research Council: Aids to the Examination of the Peripheral Nervous System, 2nd ed rev. (War Memorandum no. 7.) London, Her Majesty's Stationery Office, 1943.

65. Milner-Brown HS, Mellenthin M, Miller RG: Quantifying human muscle strength, endurance, and fatigue. Arch Phys Med Rehabil 67:530–535, 1986.

66. Mitchell GP: Poliomyelitis and exercise. Lancet 2:90–91, 1953.

67. Müller EA: Influence of training and of inactivity on muscle strength. Arch Phys Med Rehabil 51:449–462, 1970.

68. Müller EA, Beckmann H: Die trainierbarkeit von kindern mit gelähmten muskeln durch isometrische kontraktionen. Z Orthrop 102:139–145, 1966.

69. Munin MC, Jaweed MM, Staas WE, et al: Poliomyelitis muscle weakness: A prospective study of quadriceps strength. Arch Phys Med Rehabil 72:729–733, 1991.

70. Munsat TL, Andres P, Thibideau L: Preliminary observations on long-term muscle force changes in the post-polio syndrome. In Halstead LS, Wiechers DO (eds): Research and Clinical Aspects of the Late Effects of Poliomyelitis. Birth Defects 23(4):329–334, 1987.

71. Nelson KR: Creatine kinase and fibrillation potentials in patients with late sequelae of polio. Muscle Nerve 13:722–725, 1990.

72. Owen RR, Jones D: Polio residuals clinic: Conditioning exercise program. Orthopedics 8:882–883, 1985.

73. Packer TL, Martins I, Krefting L, Brouwer B: Activity and post-polio fatigue. Orthopedics 14:1223–1226, 1991.

74. Peach PE, Olejnik S: Effect of treatment and noncompliance on post-polio sequelae. Orthopedics 14:1199–1203, 1991.

75. Perry J, Barnes G, Gronley JK: The postpolio syndrome: An overuse phenomenon. Clin Orthop 233:145–162, 1988.

76. Pezeshkpour GH, Dalakas MC: Long-term changes in the spinal cords of patients with old poliomyelitis: Signs of continuous disease activity. Arch Neurol 45:505–508, 1988.

77. Ravits J, Hallett M, Baker M, et al: Clinical and electromyographic studies of post-poliomyelitis muscular atrophy. Muscle Nerve 13:667–674, 1990.

78. Raymond M (with contribution by Charcot JM): Paralysie essentiele de l'enfance: Atrophie musculaire consécutive. Gaz Med Fr (Paris) 4:225, 1875.

79. Rodriquez AA, Agre JC: Electrophysiologic study of the quadriceps muscles during fatiguing exercise and recovery: A comparison of symptomatic postpolios to asymptomatic postpolios and controls. Arch Phys Med Rehabil 72:993–997, 1991.

80. Rodriquez AA, Agre JC: Physiologic parameters and perceived exertion with local muscle fatigue in postpolio subjects. Arch Phys Med Rehabil 72:305–308, 1991.

81. Rohmert W: Ermittlung von Erholungspausen für statische Arbeit des Menschen. Int Z Angew Physiol 18:123–164, 1960.

82. Russell WR, Fischer-Williams M: Recovery of muscular strength after poliomyelitis. Lancet 1:330–333, 1954.

83. Saltin B, Blomqvist G, Mitchell JH, et al: Response to exercise after bed rest and after training: Longitudinal study of adaptive changes in oxygen transport and body composition. Circulation 38(Suppl 7):1–78, 1968.

84. Simonson E: Physiology of Work Capacity and Fatigue. Springfield, IL, Charles C Thomas, 1971.

85. Thompson RT, Barton PM, Marsh GD, Cameron MGP: Post-polio fatigue: A ^{31}P magnetic resonance spectroscopy investigation. Orthopedics 14:1263–1267, 1991.

86. Thompson RT, Gravelle D, Hahn A, Driedger AA: The biochemical heterogeneity of chronic fatigue: A^{31}P NMRS investigation [abstract 886]. Presented at the annual meeting, Society of Magnetic Resonance in Medicine, 1990.

87. Tomlinson BE, Irving D: The number of limb motor neurons in the human lumbosacral cord throughout life. J Neurol Sci 34:213–219, 1977.

88. Trojan DA, Gendron D, Cashman NR: Electrophysiology and electrodiagnosis of the post-polio motor unit. Orthopedics 14:1353–1361, 1991.

89. Van Linge B: The response of muscle to strenuous exercise: An experimental study in the rat. J Bone Joint Surg 44B:711–721, 1962.

90. Waring WP, Davidoff G, Werner R: Serum creatine kinase in the post-polio population. Am J Phys Med Rehabil 68:86–90, 1989.

91. Wiechers DO: Pathophysiology and late changes of the motor unit after poliomyelitis. In Halstead LS, Wiechers DO (eds): Late Effects of Poliomyelitis. Miami, Symposia Foundation, 1985, pp. 91–94.

92. Wiechers DO, Hubbell SL: Late changes in the motor unit after acute poliomyelitis. Muscle Nerve 4:524–528, 1981.

93. Woodwell DA: Office visits to internists, 1989. Adv Data 209:1–11, 1992.

94. Young GR: Energy conservation, occupational therapy, and the treatment of post-polio sequelae. Orthopedics 14:1233–1239, 1991.

95. Zochodne DW, Thompson RT, Driedger AA, et al: Metabolic changes in human muscle denervation: Topical ^{31}P NMR spectroscopy studies. Magn Reson Med 7:373–383, 1988.

5

Differential Diagnosis and Prognosis

ANTHONY J. WINDEBANK, MD

A number of different terms have been used to describe the late effects of polio: post-polio syndrome, post-polio progressive muscular atrophy, and the late sequelae of paralytic polio. Although each of these titles has its merits, a number of cautions should be addressed. The most important is the avoidance of attaching an all-inclusive label to an individual patient that prevents further diagnostic consideration. Broadly stated, not everyone who had polio and now has a medical problem has post-polio syndrome. The second caution is that the designation of a "syndrome" implies a cluster of symptoms and signs that are relatively homogeneous within the defined population. As discussed in this chapter, this is not the case in individuals who had polio in the past.

Extensive clinical experience at referral centers and in population-based studies suggests that there are at least three distinct symptom complexes. The first and probably most common type of difficulty involves the gradual onset, in the fourth or fifth decade, of use-related muscle pain and fatigue. These patients often complain of weakness, but close questioning reveals that this is not weakness of specific muscle groups but rather a component of the fatigue. The second type of difficulty involves degenerative joint disease or other mechanical joint or ligamentous problems caused by chronic use with inadequately stabilized joints. This is particularly true for weight-bearing joints of the axial skeleton and lower limbs and for the shoulders. The third and probably very rare type of problem involves progressive weakness and atrophy of specific muscle groups, leading to progressive loss of neuromuscular function. Because the prognosis and therapeutic approaches to these types of disorders are different, it is very important to distinguish carefully between them. As is discussed in this chapter, it is essential for each patient to evaluate carefully the cause of his or her individual symptoms so that a rational approach to therapy may be instituted.

DIAGNOSIS

One of the more difficult challenges facing the physician evaluating an individual with the late sequelae of polio is to establish the original diagnosis of polio and to determine the extent of disease. For virtually all patients presenting to physicians in developed countries, the original illness would have occurred at least 40 years ago. In our population-based study, the average age at which subjects had polio was 9 years and their average age in 1993 was 55.[20] Apart from individuals in special studies, virtually no one has records of their original illness, and many have limited childhood memories of the extent of disease. Polio was a reportable disease in most states, so it is possible for most individuals to access state records about certainty of diagnosis. However, because of the lack of efficient data-retrieval systems, this is a practical impossibility for most patients. Many social factors were influencing the diagnosis of polio in the 30s, 40s, and 50s. The disease occurred in epidemics which engendered fear in families with children and in health care providers. "Polio insurance" was an extra policy that could be purchased to provide for medical care in the event of contracting polio. These factors pressured physicians to establish a diagnosis of polio in patients with a variety of chronic or other neurologic handicaps. We have seen clear-cut cases of cerebral palsy and spina bifida that fall into this category.

The second part of establishing the original diagnosis of polio involves the distinction between paralytic and nonparalytic cases. This distinction is important because there is no credible evidence of any late-onset sequelae being related to nonparalytic polio. It has been estimated by us and others that the ratio of paralytic to nonparalytic cases is somewhere between 1:1 and 1:3. A major difficulty was the distinction between nonparalytic polio and any other viral infection. Cerebrospinal fluid examination was helpful in supporting the diagnosis but was not performed routinely in nonparalytic cases. However, because the major implications for late sequelae involve the paralytic disease, it is not critical to distinguish between nonparalytic polio and other childhood diseases. The more important distinction is the presence of a credible history of weakness due to polio. Severe back and limb pain and muscle spasms may have confounded the diagnosis of paralysis during the acute illness. This was recognized in diagnostic criteria set out in 1948 by the National Conference on Recommended Practices for the Control of Poliomyelitis (Ann Arbor, Michigan) (Table 1).

Their last criterion, "demonstrable muscle weakness or paralysis," was qualified: "Paralytic cases are defined as those in whom definite weakness or paralysis has been detected and has persisted during at least two examinations made at an interval of at least several hours. Results of an examination for paralysis of muscles of the extremities or trunk may be very unreliable during the period of muscle tenderness or spasm."

As discussed earlier, it is also important to rule out other causes of paralysis. Virtually no patients had electrophysiological testing during the acute illness. Because of the nature of the reinnervation process, electromyographic (EMG) testing now can almost always demonstrate whether an individual had significant involvement of the neurons supplying testable muscles.

The next important part of the clinical history is to determine the anatomic location and extent of original paralysis. Once again, patient memory may not be completely reliable. In recent studies,[19,20] we have compared a patient's memory of the original location of paralysis with the contemporaneous neurologic record. Commonly, individuals do not remember limbs that were less significantly involved. For example, individ-

---

TABLE 1. Diagnostic Criteria of Paralytic Poliomyelitis (1948)

Include three or more of the following:

1. History compatible with poliomyelitis

2. Fever

3. Stiff neck and/or stiff back

4. 10–500 cells/ml of spinal fluid taken during the acute or early convalescent period of the disease

5. Spinal fluid protein elevated above the normal limits

6. Demonstrable muscle weakness or paralysis.

uals with complete paralysis of the right arm may not remember mild to moderate weakness of the left arm. This has implications if they are now noticing increased difficulty in the left arm upon which they rely because of a plegic right upper limb. The important negative corollary that we have found is that progressive weakness does not occur in limbs uninvolved by the original illness.

After establishing as clearly as possible the nature and extent of the original disease, it is then important to delineate the history of present difficulties. Particular attention must be paid to differentiating between weakness of specific muscles, global fatigue, and limitation of use of muscles due to pain. All of these symptoms occur frequently in patients who had polio. Differentiation of the different components is critical for designing rational therapy for the individual patients.

DIFFERENTIAL DIAGNOSIS

Most individuals who had polio and are now presenting with increasing difficulties will have complaints involving fatigue, pain, and weakness. The cause of each should be evaluated separately and not aggregated into a single diagnosis of post-polio syndrome. After separation of each symptom, the relationship to the original polio can be considered.

WEAKNESS

It is critical to distinguish initially between specific muscle weakness, easy fatigability of individual muscles, decreased muscle use because of pain, and global fatigue. Asking about specific tasks that could be done in the past may help. For example, "Can you climb stairs in the same way as before?" If not, is the limitation due to knee pain, weakness of muscle, shortness of breath, or other? This is one of the most challenging parts of taking an accurate history in the patient who had polio. If new weakness is identified, then the time course distribution and relationship to other symptoms are critical for evaluation. This is especially true for individuals who had polio than for others complaining of weakness. When it comes to examining the patient, most will have residua from the original disease, and distinguishing this from "new" weakness may not be possible on the basis of the examination alone.

From our population-based and clinic-based studies, we have found that patients with old polio have more trouble with leg function. The most common difficulty is associated with decreasing knee stability. A residually weak quadriceps muscle, which in the past could stabilize the knee joint during weight-bearing, can now no longer do so. It is relatively uncommon for individuals with old polio to complain of progressive weakness in the upper limbs.

In those with progressive weakness, several differential diagnoses should be considered. Entrapment neuropathies are probably more common in persons who had polio. These include common unrelated entrapments, such as median neuropathy at the wrist (carpal tunnel syndrome) and entrapments specifically related to having had polio. A list of the possibilities that we have seen is set out in Table 2.

Entrapments also include roots at the vertebral level. Because of scoliosis or more rapidly advancing degenerative joint disease, individuals with polio are more prone to disc-related disease producing specific cervical or lumbosacral radiculopathies. This may be a gradual encroachment rather than an acute disc herniation. In this case, radicular pain may be less prominent.

Other unrelated neuromuscular diseases should also be considered in these individuals, who are usually over 50. These include peripheral neuropathy, myasthenia gravis, polymyositis, and muscular dystrophy. We have seen each of these masquerading as "post-polio syndrome." Clinical features may help to differentiate, as may the special investigations set out in the following section.

Other central nervous system disorders may present as weakness in the 50+ age group. These include Parkinson's disease and amyotrophic lateral

TABLE 2. Entrapment Neuropathy Seen in Persons with Polio and Related to the Residua of the Paralytic Disease

Nerve Entrapment	Cause
Ulnar nerve in hand (Guyan's canal)	Increased pressure from a cane on the heel of the hand
Ulnar nerve at elbow	Leaning on the elbow for more support in wheelchair or during transfers
Brachial plexus (especially lower trunk)	Increasing axillary crutch weight-bearing Increasing pressure in axilla from rigid body support used to support scoliotic trunk
Peroneal nerve at knee	Leg positioning in wheelchair or inappropriately fitted knee or leg brace

sclerosis. The relationship of the latter to previous polio has been contro-versial. The present weight of evidence is strongly against any relationship between antecedent polio and the development of a progressive motor neuron disease.[1–4,6,9,10,14,16]

A final factor that may contribute significantly to an apparent increase in limb weakness is weight gain. This weight gain is caused by several fac-tors, including decreased activity with age accelerated by limb weakness. This problem is greatest in patients with residual leg weakness. In our clinic referral-base patients, all patients who complained of increasing leg weakness, and for which no other cause was found, had experienced a 10–35-lb weight gain. The cause-and-effect relationship of the cycle be-tween decreased activity, increased weight, and decreased weight-bearing potential is complex, but there can be no doubt that the increased me-chanical burden of carrying extra weight contributes to the decreased abil-ity to walk. It was of note that in our population-based study[19] over a 5-year interval, patients remained stable from a neuromuscular point of view, and there was no significant change in weight of the group (Fig. 1A). On the other hand, the frequency of symptoms did not relate to weight gain in this population (Fig. 1B).

FATIGUE

There are two aspects to the symptom of fatigue: global fatigue or tired-ness and early fatigability of specific muscle groups. Weak muscles, due to any cause, are likely to fatigue with repetitive mechanical tasks more rapidly than normal muscles. However, this has been extremely difficult to demonstrate directly in the absence of specific neuromuscular junction diseases, such as myasthenia gravis. It has thus been difficult to tell whether muscle groups that are residually weak from polio have more or less endurance than normal muscles. Similarly, it has been difficult to demonstrate whether this endurance changes with aging. If fatigue of spe-cific muscles is reported, this should be investigated as if the patient were complaining of increased weakness of those muscles. Particularly, atten-tion should be paid to ruling out neuromuscular junction diseases.

Global fatigue or tiredness is often reported by individuals with resid-ual polio and by patients with other significant neurologic impairments. It is a prominent symptom in patients with multiple sclerosis. The biologic basis of this fatigue is not known. It may result from the increased effort needed to perform the normal activities of daily living. Fatigue has been a prominent symptom reported by individuals with the relatively benign form of "post-polio syndrome." The *benign* nature refers to the lack of pro-gressive neuromuscular failure. The symptoms, especially fatigue, may be

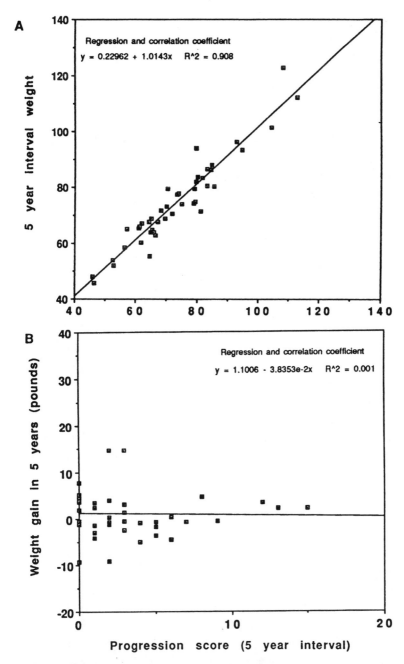

FIGURE 1. Weight change in patients with antecedent polio. Fifty patients from a population-based cohort of individuals with a documented history of paralytic polio were followed for 5 years. Weight remained stable during this period (*panel A*). There was no relationship between symptoms of fatigue, pain, weakness (progression score), and weight change (*panel B*). The progression is a tally of self-reported symptoms from a standardized questionnaire. The maximum score is 50.

very disabling. It is therefore important to rule out other causes of fatigue that are treatable by different approaches.

We have identified two independent causes of fatigue in patients who had polio. The first is *depression.* It should be stressed that in a population-based study, it was clearly demonstrated that individuals with polio were not more prone to depression and symptoms overall did not correlate with depression.[20] However, a patient with preceding polio is not protected from depression. Both reactive and endogenous components may be active as in any other individual. Reactive components may relate specifically to perceived loss of function with advancing age, especially late middle years. Individuals who had polio as a child have usually spent most of their life achieving at a high physical level to compensate for muscle weakness. This is exemplified by the pride many felt during childhood recovery as they were able to shed crutches, canes, and braces. The prospect of read-opting assistive devices may be profoundly depressing.

The second independent cause of fatigue is *sleep apnea* or other *sleep disturbance.* Sleep apnea should be suspected in anyone who complains of daytime sleepiness, snoring, morning headache, and confusion. It should additionally be suspected in persons with polio who have impaired residual respiratory function or significant weight gain. Those taking hypnotics or narcotics are particularly at risk. Sleep studies, as described later, can identify these patients and guide therapy. Therapeutic approaches to nonspecific fatigue also are discussed in the following sections.

The final point to consider is that fatigue may be a symptom of an unrelated systemic or metabolic disease. Examples such as anemia, cancer, hypothyroidism, heart failure, and diabetes all occur with increasing frequency as age progresses. Accompanying systemic symptoms should lead to appropriate separate evaluation.

PAIN

Evaluation of pain is entirely dependent on clinical history given by the patient; there is no other way it can be evaluated, and the patient's description of pain should be carefully and attentively considered. Character and location of pain together with history of onset and relationship to activity usually lead to an understanding of the origin of the pain. Both nerve entrapments and degenerative joint disease may occur more frequently in persons with antecedent polio. Those with significant residual, axial,or lower limb muscle weakness are particularly prone to degenerative joint disease in weight-bearing joints of the spine and legs. This is true for all aging individuals but may be particularly troublesome for those with residual leg weakness for two reasons. Some joints may have been poorly stabilized and used with suboptimal mechanical characteristics and geometry for many years. This may cause excessive stress and wear to cartilage as a result of uneven or unusual weight distribution. An example would be increased recurvatum of the knee. The second factor operating in those with residual weakness is that a normal limb may have compensated for a weak limb and consequently have suffered excessive wear over many years.

Muscle pain may also be a prominent feature for those with the benign form of "post-polio syndrome." Pain may be described as deep and aching, superficial and burning, or a combination of both. It is often present in many muscles, especially those of the limb girdles, spine, and proximal limbs. The pain often begins insidiously and moves from limb to limb. It occurs irregularly but is present most days. Most commonly, it does not occur with activity but is more troublesome during the evening or night of days that have involved more physical activity. Pain is worsened by psychological stress and may significantly limit activity. The pain has many characteristics of myofascial pain syndrome or fibromyalgia.[17] The cause of this pain is unknown but probably multifactorial. One factor may be chronic muscle overuse related to compensation for weakness. In some cases, this can be identified by history and therapy directed accordingly.

STUDIES TO EVALUATE POST-POLIO SYNDROME

The emphasis of the preceding discussion has been the individuality of patients and their difficulties. This individuality and a specific differential diagnosis must guide the special laboratory tests. The types of tests we have found useful are set out in Table 3. The focus of the testing algorithm is:

1. Establish the original diagnosis of polio
2. Evaluate the extent and severity of the original disease and its residua
3. Define the differential diagnosis of the present symptom complex
4. Direct tests to exclude other independent causes
5. If no other disease is found, establish a quantified baseline of function.

ESTABLISH THE ORIGINAL DIAGNOSIS OF POLIO

As discussed earlier, establishing the original diagnosis of polio may be difficult because of the lack of original medical records and the patient's poor

TABLE 3. Approaches to Laboratory Diagnosis in Patients with Antecedent Polio

Test	Indication
EMG/NCV	Evaluate residual of motor neuron disease to help establish original diagnosis and extent of disease Exclude other causes of neuromuscular impairment (e.g., radiculopathy, entrapment, peripheral neuropathy, neuromuscular junction disease, polymyositis) Establish quantitative and objective baseline of neuromuscular function
Quantitative isometric muscle-strength testing	Establish quantitative baseline of muscle strength in selected groups of muscles
Pulmonary function testing	Assess extent of present neuromuscular breathing capacity (inspiratory and expiratory pressures and maximal voluntary ventilation); baseline and impairment as basis of fatigue Exclude other respiratory problems (e.g., chronic obstructive lung disease)
Overnight oximetry (portable or telemetric)	Assess possibility of nocturnal hypoxia
Formal sleep studies	If history and oximetry suggest significant nocturnal hypoxia
Radiographs of joints	Assess extent of degenerative joint disease Assess geometry of weight-bearing joints when loaded and unloaded Assess stability of past fusions or other orthopedic procedures
Creatine kinase in blood	May be indicator of more active loss of neuromuscular function in some patients High values may indicate other muscular disorders (e.g., dystrophy polymyositis)
MMPI	Screening for occult depression
Special neuraxis imaging studies (MRI, CT of head or spine)	Only to rule out specific diseases indicated by history or examination (e.g., spinal stenosis)
Other blood tests and imaging studies	To rule out systemic diseases as indicated by history and examination (e.g., hypothyroidism, anemia, diabetes).

Abbreviations: NCV = nerve conduction velocity; MMPI = Minnesota Multiphasic Personality Inventory; MRI = magnetic resonance imaging; CT = computed tomography.

memory of a childhood disease. The neurophysiologic examination can be very helpful for this purpose. Sensory nerve conduction studies should be normal. Abnormalities, if reliably demonstrated, must be due to a second and independent cause. There should be no evidence of sensory involvement from the original disease nor from late progression of polio in any form. Focal sensory abnormality should prompt a search for local nerve compression; widespread sensory abnormalities, for a more diffuse cause of peripheral nerve disease.

Motor nerve conduction velocity (NCV) should be normal unless the evoked amplitude of the compound muscle action potential (CMAP) is very low. CMAP may be reduced secondary to loss of motor units. The pattern of CMAP reduction should approximate the pattern of clinical involvement. Needle EMG examination is most useful. During the acute illness, motor neurons in the spinal cord were lost, and muscle fibers were left without innervation. During the recovery process, reinnervation occurred by collateral sprouting from the distal axons of surviving motor neurons. This only occurred within muscles whose motor neuron pool had been attacked by the virus. As a result, large and complex motor units are seen within these muscles, but uninvolved muscles remain normal. Motor units may have become very large and in severely affected muscles; individual surviving motor neurons may have reached the upper limit of their ability to reinnervate muscle fibers. It has been suggested that as a result, there may be an ongoing dynamic process of remodeling where individual muscle fibers are losing their extended axon terminals and other fibers are reinnervated by sprouting.[5] Because of this process and, perhaps, because of the extended length of terminal sprouts, the safety factor for neuromuscular transmission may have decreased. Electromyographically, this may manifest as variability in the morphology of an individual motor unit potential (MUP) during repeated firing.

This may be part of the physiologic basis of fatigue.[5,8] A shift in the equilibrium of this remodeling process toward net denervation may be the basis of progressive weakness in individuals with post-polio progressive muscular atrophy. This concept both has and has not been confirmed in our population-based study.[19] Because the capacity for reinnervation in more severely affected muscles may be exceeded by the number of denervated muscle fibers, some fibers may not have been reinnervated. These atrophic and orphaned fibers continue to produce fibrillation potentials indefinitely. Typically, these fibrillation potentials are very small spikes. These chronic, small fibrillation potentials may be seen in the context of any process which produced denervation many years previously (E. Lambert, personal communication). The dynamic remodeling process may produce more recently denervated fibers and higher amplitude fibrillation potentials. In our experience, the frequency of larger fibrillation potentials is one of the useful indicators of progressive denervation and corresponds most closely to symptoms of progressive weakness. Finally, the interference pattern will reflect loss of motor units so that rate of MUP recruitment is increased in affected muscles.

In summary, observation of MUP morphology and firing pattern will confirm whether limb muscles were involved with a previous motor neuron disease and may give clues about the etiology of symptoms. The distribution will reflect the distribution of involvement of the original disease, although the sensitivity for detection of EMG changes may show broader involvement than was suspected clinically.

The major differential diagnosis for this pattern of EMG changes is progressive spinal muscular atrophy, especially the chronic, slowly progressive form of the disease. The symmetry of the latter process and the clinical history may serve to differentiate these processes. The rare possibility of independent SMA superimposed on old polio may be indistinguishable. The EMG abnormalities will reliably distinguish a new, primarily myopathic process. A normal, adequately performed EMG excludes a history of paralytic polio affecting examined muscles and, therefore, may help to eliminate this diagnosis in individuals with chronic muscle pain and fatigue not related to old polio.

EVALUATE THE EXTENT AND SEVERITY OF THE ORIGINAL DISEASE AND ITS RESIDUA

The EMG examination, as discussed, is the single most reliable test in this process. Two additional studies have been helpful for us, in addition to careful clinical examination. Measurement of *isometric muscle strength*, which is now available in many physical medicine or orthopedic departments, measures force generated across a joint. With good patient cooperation and carefully controlled stabilization of limbs, reproducible measurements may be produced. If available, in the individual laboratory, these results may be compared with age; gender; and habitus-matched population norms. This extends the clinical examination but may be a more sensitive indicator of small changes over time. The experienced operator can usually distinguish between submaximal subject effort and neuromuscular-based weakness. The importance of careful attention to measurement techniques cannot be over-stressed.[18]

Measurement of *pulmonary function* also serves as a baseline and assessment of extent of involvement. We have found the static pressures (maximal inspiratory pressure and maximal expiratory pressure or bugle pressures) and the maximal voluntary ventilation in 2 minutes to be the most useful indicators. Forced vital capacity is also useful as a repeated long-term measure of pulmonary function. Dynamic airflow tests (forced-expiratory volume in 1 minute/forced vital capacity ratio, etc.) are most useful in excluding primary obstructive lung disease or other independent causes of respiratory symptoms. Overnight oximetry or formal study may be required for evaluation of those with symptoms suggestive of nocturnal respiratory failure or sleep apnea.

DEFINE THE DIFFERENTIAL DIAGNOSIS OF THE PRESENT SYMPTOM COMPLEX

The differential diagnosis is the most critical part of the integrated clinical and laboratory approach to the patient. Careful evaluation of symptoms, in association with the electrophysiologic studies, allows very specific direction of other laboratory tests. This is best illustrated with a brief example. A person with a history of paralytic polio involving all four limbs presents with progressive left hand weakness. Clinical examination is compatible with old polio but cannot distinguish whether the left hand intrinsic muscle atrophy is new or old. Electrophysiologic studies suggest compression of the ulnar nerve in Guyan's canal in the hand. Cause is identified as increasing weight-bearing pressure through the heel of the hand on a cane, and therapy is appropriately directed.

DIRECT TESTS TO EXCLUDE OTHER INDEPENDENT CAUSES

The process described above might lead to a location of entrapment and nerve trunk or root compression. Imaging studies may then be required to exclude compressive lesions. Alternatively, the differential diagnosis may be directed to systemic causes of fatigue and weakness, such as hypothyroidism or anemia.

IF NO OTHER DISEASE IS FOUND, ESTABLISH A QUANTIFIED BASELINE OF FUNCTION

We have found the clinical and electrophysiologic examination, the quantitative evaluation of isometric muscle strength, and pulmonary function tests to be the most useful markers of function in polio. Repeat measurements over intervals of years will document change and yield information about the cause of change. In repeated evaluations over time in individual subjects, it is important to keep an open mind about the etiology of new symptoms.

PROGNOSIS

Estimates of the frequency with which polio survivors develop late progressive problems have been difficult to ascertain. When first reports of progressive, late-onset weakness were published,[15] it appeared that this was a rare entity. However, many reports appearing during the last 10 years have suggested that a variety of difficulties may be occurring with much greater frequency than expected. In order to gain more insight into this question, we utilized the resources of the Rochester and Olmsted County, Minnesota, database. This database contains all medical information about the residents of the county in southeastern Minnesota in which the Mayo Clinic is situated. More importantly, the information has been stored in retrievable records with coded diagnosis for all medical contacts. Using this database, we were able to identify all residents of this county who suffered from paralytic poliomyelitis between 1935 and 1960. The definition of paralytic polio was that used by the National Conference of Recommended Practices for the control of poliomyelitis described earlier in this chapter.

Using this definition and the original medical records from the time of the acute illness, 300 individuals were identified who fulfilled these criteria. The completeness of ascertainment was checked by comparing with state records; reporting of polio to the State of Minnesota was mandatory. Of the 300 individuals, 298 were traced at the beginning of the study in 1986. A telephone survey indicated that about 21% of these individuals might be experiencing some form of late progressive difficulty.[7] In order to understand the cause of these symptoms, we selected a cohort of 50 individuals for a prospective study. These 50 individuals were representative of the survivors. The characteristics of the original illness, severity, and distribution of paralysis were similar between the study cohort and the whole group of survivors.[20] The 50 subjects were not chosen on the basis of any new difficulties but because they had paralytic polio and were Olmsted County residents when they had their acute illness. Individuals who had polio elsewhere and later moved to the county were not included.

The cohort of 50 survivors were then studied in detail using a structured history questionnaire, scored neurologic examination, detailed electrophysiological studies, isometric muscle strength measurement, pulmonary function tests, psychological inventories, and timed tests of function, such as gait and upper limb dexterity. These tests were then repeated 5 years later to assess stability or progression within this cohort.

The characteristics of the cohort have been described in detail.[20] The mean age at which they suffered acute polio was 9 years and their mean age at the time of entry into the study was 50 years (range, 35–71 years). This was therefore not a population of advanced aged individuals. The 41-year interval between acute illness and time of follow-up was characteristic of the population thought to be at risk for developing post-polio syndrome.

In this cohort, at the time of first study in 1986, about 60% had at least one of the symptoms of pain, fatigue, or progressive weakness. In only 20% was this of sufficient severity to necessitate some change in lifestyle or activities of daily living.[20] The types of changes ranged from the need for additional bracing to taking early retirement because of inability to walk long distances. Over the 5-year prospective study, the number of individuals with some complaints remained stable at approximately 60%, and the distribution of the types and frequency of complaints also remained stable (Fig. 2).

Measures of function in the cohort were remarkably stable over the 5-year prospective observation period. The time taken to walk 100 ft actually improved slightly from 27.6 S (SD, 7.5 s) to 23.6 S (SD, 5.3 s). This difference, although small, was statistically highly significant (p < 0.0001, 2-tailed paired t-test). Tests of upper limb dexterity (Minnesota Rate of Manipulation Test for placing, turning, and displacing) did not change significantly during the observation period.

Scored neurologic examination was similarly stable.[20] This score is 0 in a normal individual and 268 in an individual who has complete paralysis of all motor functions and loss of all limb reflexes and sensation. At the height of acute illness, the mean score in the cohort was 31 (range, 1–140.5). At the first time point in the prospective study, the mean was 20.3 (range, 0–120.5) and had improved to 17.1 (range, 0–121) after the 5-year interval. This small difference was statistically significant (p = 0.0036). The stability of this observation using linear regression analysis was quite striking. The slope of the second disability score against the first was 0.998 with a high correlation coefficient (r^2 = 0.953).

Electrophysiological variables were also well preserved. The most reproducible comparison of overall motor function is the summated CMAP. Using bilateral median and peroneal CMAP amplitudes, the mean at first observation was 27.7 mV (SD, 10.1 mV), and 5 years later was 29.3 mV (SD, 11.2 mV). This small trend toward improvement was not statistically significant (p = 0.195) but was in the same direction as the walking and total neurologic disability scores.

Because this stability was counter to current opinion, we looked at the data in a number of other ways. We were first concerned whether a limb or muscle that was not involved by the original disease could later experience impairment of neuromuscular function. We had detailed neurologic examinations on all subjects at the time of their acute illness, in 1986–87 and 1991–92. We were thus able to ask whether any muscles were affected in later years that were not involved during the original illness. Of 2,700 muscles examined in the 50 patients, only 4 examples were found. In each case, the changes were small. This could certainly be accounted for by the original examiners missing a weak muscle in an acutely ill child. The over-

FIGURE 2. Stability of symptom numbers in patients with polio. *Panel A* shows the distribution of progressive scores (*see* Fig. 1) in 1986–87, and *panel B*, in the same 50 patients 5 years later.

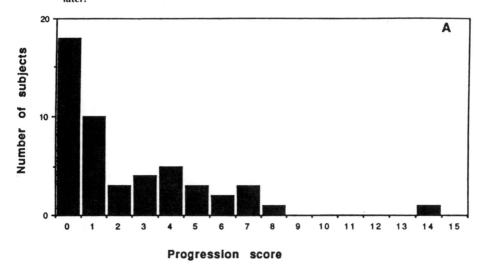

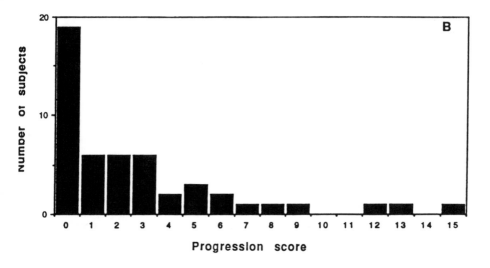

whelming conclusion was that if a limb was not involved with the original disease process, it would not subsequently develop difficulties on a neuromuscular basis. This does not exclude the possibility that a normal limb that has compensated for a weak one for many years may not develop degenerative joint disease more rapidly than expected.

The second area of concern was that since we were analyzing a whole population of individuals with a spectrum of severity of disease, significant changes in affected limbs might be statistically lost in the majority of normal limbs. We, therefore, reanalyzed our data by separating all normal limbs from those affected by the paralytic process. To do this, we considered each subject as five separate "limbs" (2 arms, 2 legs, and the bulbar musculature). We then looked at every "limb" separately and determined whether it was involved by the original paralytic disease. We then compared changes in the control limbs, which had never shown clinical evidence of disease involvement, with the paretic limbs which had been involved. There were 115 "control" limbs and 135 "paretic" limbs. For these limbs, we compared the changes in neurologic disability score, isometric muscle strength, CMAP amplitude of the muscles measured in that limb and number of motor unit potentials estimated in a muscle in that limb. There were no significant differences between these variables in the two types of limbs.

A final concern was that the assessment tools used to measure changes over 5 years were not significantly sensitive. Because of extensive population-based studies of diabetics in this same population, we believe this is not the case.[11] These same instruments have been highly effective in detecting the presence and documenting the progression of diabetic neuropathy over a similar time interval.

In summary, all of our measures of neuromuscular function demonstrated stability in this group of subjects. This demonstrates that deteriorating neuromuscular function is not widespread in this population-based study of individuals who had paralytic polio. This does not mean that "post-polio syndrome" does not exist. Complaints of limb pain and aching, weakness, and fatigue were common in this population (Table 4).[20] Causes other than neuromuscular deterioration must be sought to explain these. Our studies were not designed to detect or measure these, but we believe that degenerative joint disease and overuse syndromes are a major contributor to these symptoms. This is an important conclusion because effective treatment strategies are available in physical medicine and orthopedic disciplines to manage this type of problem.

Similarly, our data do not exclude a small group of patients who may have progressive neuromuscular impairment. These individuals are of the

TABLE 4. New Difficulties Experienced by Subjects with Prior Paralytic Polio*

		Patients	
Symptom	No.	Requiring New Aids (n)	Changing Activities (n)
Fatigue alone	2	1	0
Pain alone	7†	0	1
Pain and fatigue	1	1	0
Weakness alone	4	0	0
Weakness and pain	9	2	0
Weakness and fatigue	2	1	0
Weakness, pain, and fatigue	7	2	1
No new symptoms	18	0	0

*Types of complaints reported by 32 of 50 subjects with paralytic polio.
Twenty-one complained of some new weakness. In 7 subjects, the new symptoms necessitated the use of new aids to daily living, and in 2 different cases, the symptoms had led to lifestyle changes.
†All 7 complained of nonradiating lumbar or cervical pain.
From Windebank AJ, Litchy WJ, Daube JR, et al: Late effects of paralytic poliomyelitis in Olmsted County, Minnesota. *Neurology* 41:501–507, 1991; with permission.

type described by Mulder[15] and probably account for those with deteriorating neuromuscular function observed in post-polio clinic-based studies.[8] In personal referral practice, we have seen similar patients. In this sample of referred patients, the most common difficulty is decreased weight-bearing capacity and inability to stabilize the knee joint. This usually occurs because of increased quadriceps weakness, although internal derangement of the knee joint secondary to degenerative changes may contribute. The increased quadriceps weakness occurs in a muscle that was probably functioning at borderline and was just able to stabilize the joint. A minor loss of muscle function produces a major change in gait if the knee cannot be stabilized in weight-bearing extension. Whether this increased weakness is due to overuse, natural attrition of motor neurons with age,[12,13] or the remodeling process described earlier is unknown. Evidence of progressive neuromuscular failure in upper limbs of patients with polio is very rare, and when this occurs, separate independent causes should be sought.

ACKNOWLEDGMENTS

The secretarial assistance of Ms. Linda A. Goldbeck is gratefully acknowledged. Parts of the data reviewed in this chapter were presented at the New York Academy of Sciences meeting in Bethesda, Maryland, April 1994, and at the 46th Annual Meeting of the American Academy of Neurology in Washington, DC, May 1994.

REFERENCES

1. Alter M, Kurland LT, Molgaard CA: Late progressive muscular atrophy and antecedent poliomyelitis. Adv Neurol 36:303–309, 1982.

2. Armon C, Daube JR, Windebank AJ, Kurland LT: How frequently does classic amyotrophic lateral sclerosis develop in survivors of poliomyelitis? Neurology 40:172–174, 1990.

3. Brahic M, Smith RA, Gibbs CJ Jr, et al: Detection of picornavirus sequences in nervous tissue of amyotrophic lateral sclerosis and control patients. Ann Neurol 18:337–343, 1985.

4. Brown S, Patten BM: Post-polio syndrome and amyotrophic lateral sclerosis: A relationship more apparent than real. Birth Defects 23(4):83–98, 1987.

5. Cashman NR, Maselli R, Wollmann RL, et al: Late denervation in patients with antecedent paralytic poliomyelitis. N Engl J Med 317:7–12, 1987.

6. Chiò A, Meineri P, Tribolo A, Schiffer D: Risk factors in motor neuron disease: A case-control study. Neuroepidemiology 10:174–184, 1991.

7. Codd MB, Mulder DW, Kurland LT, et al: Poliomyelitis in Rochester, Minnesota, 1935–1955: Epidemiology and long-term sequelae: A preliminary report. In Halstead LS, Wiechers DO, (eds): Late Effects of Poliomyelitis. Miami, Symposia Foundation, 1985, pp 121–134

8. Dalakas MC, Elder G, Hallett M, et al: A long-term follow-up study of patients with post-poliomyelitis neuromuscular symptoms. N Engl J Med 314:959–963, 1986.

9. Deapen DM, Henderson BE: A case-control study of amyotrophic lateral sclerosis. Am J Epidemiol 123:790–799, 1986.

10. den Hartog Jager WA, Hanlo PW, Ansink BJJ, Vermeulen MBM: Results of a questionnaire in 100 ALS patients and 100 control cases. Clin Neurol Neurosurg 89:37–41, 1987.

11. Dyck PJ, Kratz KM, Lehman KA, et al: The Rochester Diabetic Neuropathy Study: Design, criteria for types of neuropathy, selection bias, and reproducibility of neuropathic tests. Neurology 41:799–807, 1991.

12. Kawamura Y, Dyck PJ: Lumbar motoneurons of man: III. The number and diameter distribution of large- and intermediate-diameter cytons by nuclear columns. J Neuropathol Exp Neurol 36:956–963, 1977.

13. Kawamura Y, O'Brien P, Okazaki H, Dyck PJ: Lumbar motoneurons of man: II. The number and diameter distribution of large- and intermediate-diameter cytons in "motoneuron columns" of spinal cord of man. J Neuropathol Exp Neurol 36:861–870, 1977.

14. Miller JR, Guntaka RV, Myers JC: Amyotrophic lateral sclerosis: Search for poliovirus by nucleic acid hybridization. Neurology 30:884–886, 1980.

15. Mulder DW, Rosenbaum RA, Layton DD Jr: Late progression of poliomyelitis or forme fruste amyotrophic lateral sclerosis? Mayo Clin Proc 47:756–761, 1972.

16. Roos RP, Viola MV, Wollmann R, et al: Amyotrophic lateral sclerosis with antecedent poliomyelitis. Arch Neurol 37:312–313, 1980.

17. Thompson JM: Tension myalgia as a diagnosis at the Mayo Clinic and its relationship to fibrositis, fibromyalgia, and myofascial pain syndrome. Mayo Clin Proc 65:1237–1248, 1990.

18. Windebank AJ: Clinical evaluation of motor function. In PJ Dyck, PK Thomas, AK Asbury, et al (eds): Diabetic Neuropathy. Philadelphia, W.B. Saunders, 1987, pp 100–106

19. Windebank AJ, Daube JR, Litchy WJ, Iverson R: A population-based study of the late effects of paralytic poliomyelitis [abstract]. Neurology 44:256, 1994.

20. Windebank AJ, Litchy WJ, Daube JR, et al: Late effects of paralytic poliomyelitis in Olmsted County, Minnesota. Neurology 41:501–507, 1991.

21. Windebank AJ, Daube JR, Litchy WJ, et al: Late sequelae of paralytic poliomyelitis in Olmstead County, Minnesota. Birth Defects 23:27–38, 1987.

6

Evaluation and Management of Post-Polio Respiratory Sequelae: Noninvasive Options

JOHN R. BACH, MD

Post-poliomyelitis inspiratory, expiratory, and bulbar muscle weakness can lead to chronic alveolar hypoventilation (CAH), intercurrent pulmonary complications, and respiratory failure. There may also be a higher incidence of sleep-disordered breathing in this population. However, because of their insidious nature, respiratory symptoms are often misinterpreted and the general lack of knowledge of noninvasive respiratory muscle aids leads to inappropriate management strategies. Episodes of acute respiratory failure associated with otherwise benign respiratory tract infections (RTIs) or elective surgical procedures often punctuate an insidiously progressive course. Unnecessarily invasive evaluation and management approaches adversely affect quality of life and can increase the risk of pulmonary complications and mortality.

HISTORICAL PERSPECTIVE

Over 500,000 people were afflicted with poliomyelitis in the United States during the 35-year period from 1928—the year that the iron lung was per-   **89** fected—through 1962.[56] About 15% of patients with paralytic polio developed ventilatory failure and/or swallowing impairment.[66] In the 1952 polio epidemic in Denmark, the mortality was 94% for those with respiratory paralysis with bulbar involvement, and 28% for those with respiratory paralysis without bulbar involvement.[66] Twenty-five of 200 surviving post-poliomyelitis ventilator-assisted individuals (PVAIs) (12.5%) remained ventilator assisted. The Danes reported that overall mortality figures for PVAIs decreased from 80% to 41% in part because of more frequent use of tracheostomy.[66]

In the meantime, specialized centers in the United States were also reporting significant decreases in mortality without resorting to tracheostomy for intermittent positive pressure ventilation (IPPV) by "individualizing" patient care. From 1948 to 1952, 15–20% of 3,500 polio patients treated at Los Angeles General Hospital required ventilatory support. It was reported that general mortality decreased from 12–15% to 1948 to 2% in 1952.[57] Although many patients at Los Angeles General Hospital, particularly those with bulbar polio, had tracheostomies placed for management of secretions while they were ventilated by negative pressure body ventilators (NPBVs), in other centers where few tracheostomies were performed, mortality also decreased to about 2%.[57] Therefore, the earlier high fatality rate was not necessarily due to the inefficiency of body ventilators but to inadequate management of bulbar muscle insufficiency and aspiration.[57] Better nursing care and attention to managing airway secretions including the use of appropriate mechanical devices were factors in decreasing mortality rates.[22–25,27,89] These latter devices continue to be important for many PVAIs.[8,10,12,13,15]

The first report of late-onset post-polio ventilatory insufficiency was in 1970.[52] In 1987, Bach et al.[13] studied 75 PVAIs, of whom 31 were late onset at an average of 18 years post polio. More recently, the majority of PVAIs have been described as late onset.[10,45] Some post-paralytic poliomyelitis individuals (PPIs) who did not require ventilatory assistance during acute poliomyelitis were also now using ventilators.[10,45,58] A recent national survey of the late effects of poliomyelitis found that 42% of the respondents reported new breathing problems.[51]

PATHOPHYSIOLOGY OF LATE-ONSET PULMONARY DYSFUNCTION

Respiratory muscle weakness occurs because of the effects of aging, fatigue, and/or accelerated loss of remaining anterior horn cell collaterals on respiratory muscle. This leads to a decrease in pulmonary volumes, including vital capacity (VC), and to a decrease in maximum inspiratory and expiratory pressures and airflows. With aging, PPIs who develop late-onset ventilatory insufficiency lose VC at a rate of 60–90% greater than normal.[13,45] It is likely that PPIs in general also lose VC at accelerated rates. The resulting restrictive pulmonary syndrome is often exacerbated by the presence of scoliosis and leads to insidious ventilatory insufficiency. Hypercapnia is likely when the VC falls below 55% of predicted normal.[30] Symptoms, however, may be minimal for nonambulatory patients as gradual resetting of respiratory control centers accommodates to CAH.[8] Hypoxia, hypercapnia, and loss in VC are exacerbated when intrinsic lung disease, kyphoscoliosis, sleep-disordered breathing, or obesity complicates inspiratory muscle weakness.

Likewise, expiratory muscle weakness decreases peak cough expiratory flows (PCEF). This impairs the ability to clear airway secretions, particularly during RTIs. Airway obstruction from laryngeal muscle incompetence, from aspiration of airway secretions and food due to bulbar involvement, from vocal cord paralysis or tracheal stenosis due to previous endotracheal intubation, or for any other reason hampers expiratory muscle function and can further decrease PCEF. A history of smoking or the presence of chronic bronchorrhea for any reason further increases the tendency of patients with weak expiratory and/or bulbar musculature to develop chronic mucus plugging. Chronic mucus plugging leads to ventilation/perfusion imbalance, atelectasis, pneumonias, pulmonary scarring, and loss of lung compliance. A large mucus plug can cause sudden hypoxia and acute respiratory failure. If not properly managed, such patients may require repeated intubation, bronchoscopy, and tracheostomy. PCEFs of 5 L/s or greater are necessary for effective airway secretion and mucus clearance.[20] It is failure to attain adequate PCEFs that correlates best with the risk of pulmonary complications.

The rapid shallow breathing pattern with loss of the ability to take occasional deep inspirations (sighs) contributes to loss of pulmonary compliance, increased stiffness of the rib cage, and chronic microatelectasis.[38,44] This is also exacerbated by the presence of scoliosis. Decreased pulmonary compliance increases the work of breathing.

Sleep-disordered breathing, which is the occurrence of central or obstructive apneas and hypopneas, occurs to some degree in 37.5% of the general population older than 62 years of age.[32] A symptomatic individual with a mean of 10 or more apneas plus hypopneas per hour is said to have obstructive sleep apnea syndrome (OSAS).[48,54] There appears to be a greater incidence of sleep-disordered breathing in PPIs due both to paresis of intrinsic muscles of the larynx[57] and to damage to respiratory control centers from the encephalitic process of the primary viral infection.[55,57,79,81] Guilleminault and Motta noted a mixed obstructive-central apnea picture in 5 PPIs.[50] Steljes et al. demonstrated obstructive or mixed apneas in 7 of 8 PPIs with complaints of fatigue, muscle weakness, muscle or joint pain, sleep problems, and breathing difficulties.[87] Sleep-disordered breathing alone can result in CAH, in hypoxia, in right ventricular strain, and, when severe, in acute cardiopulmonary failure.

Arterial oxygen tensions of 10–20 mm Hg less than normal means for age signal the presence of microatelectasis in otherwise stable restrictive pulmonary syndrome patients with normal chest radiographs. Significant intrinsic lung disease is present when the PO_2 is less than 60 mm Hg in the absence of hypercapnia and reversible factors. Correction of serum acid–base balance by use of inspiratory muscle aids that normalize alveolar ventilation greatly reduces right ventricular strain.[43]

When not corrected, insidiously progressive hypercapnia leads to compensatory metabolic alkalosis. The resulting elevated central nervous system bicarbonate levels contribute to depression of the ventilatory response to hypoxia and hypercapnia. This permits worsening of CAH, and it may decrease the effectiveness of nocturnal noninvasive IPPV once that treatment modality is instituted[8] until the problem is corrected by normalizing alveolar ventilation around the clock.

RESPIRATORY EVALUATION

Patients' symptoms should not be dismissed as due to "post-polio syndrome" without an adequate evaluation of respiratory function, including sleep studies when indicated. The evaluation should take into account the patient's pulmonary history and symptomatology, VC, maximum insufflation capacity (MIC) when the VC is less than 1,500 ml, PCEF, noninvasive blood gas monitoring, and, on infrequent occasions, when the diagnosis is unclear, ambulatory polysomnography. Obesity, abdominal distention, and acute RTIs decrease both inspiratory and expiratory muscle function.[73] Arterial blood gas sampling should be used only for acutely ill patients to monitor supplemental oxygen administration after alveolar ventilation has been normalized by inspiratory muscle aids.

Post-polio symptoms and signs are said to include fatigue, headache, sleep disturbances, decreased muscle strength, muscle aches, dyspnea, cyanosis, irritability, anxiety, and depression.[61] These symptoms, however, are also characteristic of CAH and OSAS.[8] Other symptoms and signs of CAH or OSAS include hypersomnolence, poor concentration, impaired intellectual function and memory, nightmares particularly concerning breathing, decreased libido, and recent changes in body weight. Patients with impaired oropharyngeal muscle function may also complain of difficulty swallowing and managing airway secretions.[8] Partial vocal cord or glottic paralysis is a common cause for inadequate generation of PCEF. Concomitant obstructive airway disease in these middle-aged or elderly PPIs, particularly the chronic smokers, will also decrease PCEF. Evaluation of forced expiratory flows as well as PCEF should be done whenever chronic obstructive pulmonary disease (COPD) is suspected.

If the pulmonary dysfunction is primarily restrictive, then regular measurement of VC with an accurate portable spirometer is sufficient for monitoring patient progress and response to treatment. The VC should be measured in the sitting position, in the supine position, with other positional changes, and while using thoracolumbar orthoses when appropriate. If the VC is less than 1,500 ml, the MIC should be determined. The MIC is a measure of the maximum volume of air that can be held with a closed glottis. It is obtained by the air stacking of mechanical insufflations and/or by glossopharyngeal breathing (GPB).[12] The MIC is a function of pulmonary compliance and the strength of bulbar musculature. For PPIs, an MIC of at least 1,000 ml is needed to achieve adequate PCEF for airway secretion management and therefore permit optimal continued use of noninvasive aids without resort to tracheostomy or mechanical insufflation-exsufflation.[5] The MIC is also of great value in predicting GPB potential and the glossopharyngeal maximum single breath capacity (GPmaxSBC).[12]

Any patient with daytime hypercapnia or less than 50% of predicted normal supine VC should undergo oxyhemoglobin saturation (SaO_2) monitoring and possibly PCO_2 monitoring during sleep. The capnograph, which can be used to measure end-tidal PCO_2, and pulse oximeter must be capable of summarizing and printing out the data.[8,15] These studies are most conveniently performed on an ambulatory basis. Transcutaneous CO_2 sleep studies can also be done on an inpatient basis with CO_2 sensing electrodes. The diagnosis of CAH is established by the observation of nocturnal PCO_2 greater than 50 mm Hg. Without nocturnal PCO_2 data, continuous oxyhemoglobin desaturation with a mean of less than 95% for 1 hour or more during sleep in a symptomatic patient with VC of less than 50% of predicted normal is sufficient to establish the diagnosis and initiate treatment. With CAH, nocturnal hypoventilation is usually more severe than daytime hypoventilation.[18] Without concomitant central or obstructive apneas or hypopneas, nocturnal SaO_2 monitoring typically reveals a relatively smooth decrease in baseline waking SaO_2.

Although patients with severe CAH and a mean sleep SaO_2 under 90% can have many transient and often severe decreases in saturation, a saw-tooth pattern of oxyhemoglobin desaturation with more than 10 transient 4% or greater drops per hour in a symptomatic patient with relatively normal supine VC and mean SaO_2 signals the presence of sleep-disordered breathing. For symptomatic patients, oximetry studies are highly sensitive in screening for this condition.[62,90]

For symptomatic patients with supine VCs greater than 50% of predicted normal and with inconclusive nocturnal oximetry and carbon dioxide studies, the symptomatology may be explained on the basis of a combination of inspiratory muscle weakness and sleep-disordered breathing or other factors. Ambulatory polysomnography may assist in the evaluation.[82]

PULMONARY MANAGEMENT OF PPIS

Management of a restrictive pulmonary syndrome with CAH or sleep-disordered breathing should not await hospitalization for acute respiratory failure. Both sleep-disordered breathing and CAH can be reversed, respiratory control mechanisms normalized, and life quality and longevity increased with treatment that can be initiated in either the home or clinic environment. The primary goals for the appropriate patient should be to maintain normal alveolar ventilation around the clock, to provide effective clearance of airway secretions, to maintain or improve at least dynamic pulmonary compliance, and, when present, to address the factors that cause sleep-disordered breathing. PPIs may have sleep-disordered breathing, CAH, or some combination of each. There are PPIs for whom neither sleep-disordered breathing nor the restrictive pulmonary syndrome are severe enough to warrant treatment but who with both conditions require aid to maintain adequate ventilation.[13,15]

SLEEP-DISORDERED BREATHING

Any reversible conditions associated with OSAS should be identified and treated.[68,84] Otherwise, continuous positive airway pressure (CPAP) is effective for the majority of patients for whom no treatable etiological condition can be found. CPAP works as a pneumatic splint to maintain an open airway. CPAP of 5–15 cm H_2O is usually adequate. Independently varying the inspiratory (IPAP) and expiratory (EPAP) pressures with the use of bilevel positive airway pressure (Bi-PAP, Respironics Inc., Monroeville, Pennsylvania) can improve effectiveness and comfort. To optimize treatment efficacy, nocturnal recordings of SaO_2 should be made at various CPAP or Bi-PAP settings. For patients with paralytic/restrictive ventilatory insufficiency and sleep-disordered breathing, both CPAP and Bi-PAP with low IPAP/EPAP ratios may be ineffective. Either a high IPAP/EPAP ratio or the use of other portable pressure or volume-cycled ventilators for noninvasive IPPV delivered via oral, nasal, or oral-nasal patient-ventilator hose interfaces should be used. Noninvasive IPPV assists or supports the patient's ventilation and maintains upper airway patency.[8,13,15,17,31,34,50,67,87] The use of Demand Positive Airway Pressure (Medical Systems Inc., Hampton, New Hampshire), in which positive pressure varies with the airflows created during autonomous breathing, has yet to be adequately evaluated or compared with Bi-PAP in clinical settings.

Even when effective, CPAP, Bi-PAP, and noninvasive IPPV may not be tolerated due to discomfort or air leakage from an inadequately fitting CPAP mask.[89] Several of the at least seven varieties of commercially available CPAP masks should be offered to each patient.[7] Some commercially available masks can be custom molded to the patient's nose, such as SE-FAM-style masks (Fig. 1) (Lifecare Inc., Lafayette, Colorado). Such interfaces are comfortable and effective at higher pressures, but they are also

FIGURE 1. SEFAM custom-molded nosepiece for CPAP, Bi-PAP, or nasal IPPV. (Courtesy of Lifecare International Inc., Lafayette, Colorado.)

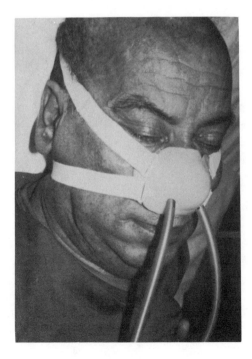

expensive and delicate, and they require frequent refabrication. Transparent, durable, custom-molded, low-profile nasal interfaces can also be prepared from a plaster moulage (Fig. 2).[70] They are comfortable and cosmetic. Various other orthotic and surgical options are also possible for OSAS patients when positive airway pressure is not well tolerated.[29,33,63,83,88] However, they may not be adequate for patients with hypercapnia.

CHRONIC ALVEOLAR HYPOVENTILATION OR CHRONIC VENTILATORY FAILURE

The symptoms of CAH are often misdiagnosed and the PPI is often suboptimally managed even when the diagnosis is established in a timely manner. Untreated PPIs with CAH may present with recurrent bouts of pneumonia and acute respiratory failure particularly during otherwise benign RTIs. Such patients are hospitalized and receive intermittent positive pressure breathing (IPPB) treatments for the delivery of bronchodilators, xanthine derivatives, and other generally ineffective medications for patients with purely restrictive pulmonary conditions. Likewise, oxygen therapy is often unnecessarily prescribed both before and after discharge.

FIGURE 2. Low-profile, transparent, custom-molded acrylic nosepiece for CPAP, Bi-PAP, or nasal IPPV.[43]

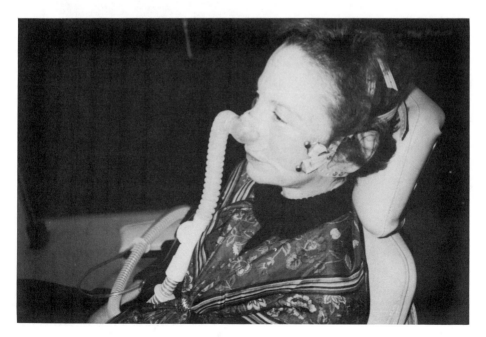

The use of long-term oxygen therapy instead of emphasis on providing maximal insufflations, optimal ventilation, and assisted coughing can worsen hypoventilation and hypercapnia. This increases microatelectasis, decreases pulmonary compliance, and can hasten the occurrence of a respiratory arrest.[8,26,45,52] For PPIs with CAH, oxygen therapy should be avoided unless significant hypoxia persists following normalization of carbon dioxide levels with the use of noninvasive inspiratory muscle aids. Since few physicians are familiar with noninvasive respiratory muscle aids, reluctant patients all too often are coerced into accepting a tracheostomy, with its potential complications and inconveniences. They often subsequently regret the decision.[1]

Ventilatory assistance or support can be provided by NPBVs—ventilators that act directly on the body— and by noninvasive IPPV methods. NPBVs create negative pressure on the chest and abdomen, causing air to flow into the lungs through the nose and mouth.[16] They include the iron lung,[41] Porta-Lung,[16] chest shell ventilator,[65,86] and negative pressure wrap ventilators.[16] These devices have been used for nocturnal ventilatory support for decades by hundreds of PVAIs.[12,13] They are inconvenient and not always effective. Travel is difficult and intimacy with a significant other may be impossible. In a small study of PPIs using NPBVs, Steljes et al. observed poor sleep quality, a high apnea hypopnea index, hypoxia, and hypercapnia.[87] Use of NPBVs is associated with obstructive sleep apneas and often severe oxyhemoglobin desaturations of uncertain clinical significance in the majority of individuals who use them.[19] The usual occurrences of heavy snoring and observed breathing difficulties often seen in unaided patients with OSAS may not be present in patients using NPBVs.[19]

Ventilators that act directly on the body include the rocking bed[49] and the intermittent abdominal pressure ventilator (IAPV). The rocking bed rocks from 15° to 30°. The rocking moves the abdominal contents, and the resulting diaphragmatic excursion assists alveolar ventilation. The rocking bed presents many of the same difficulties and inconveniences as the NPBVs and is in general less effective. The IAPV consists of an inflatable bladder in an abdominal belt. The bladder is cyclically inflated by a portable ventilator. The alternating pressure on the abdominal contents moves the diaphragm and ventilates the patient. The IAPV generally augments the patient's autonomous tidal volumes by more than 300 ml.[11] It is most effective in the sitting position at 75–80°. It is the method of choice for daytime ventilatory support for most individuals with less than one hour of ventilator-free time, because it is cosmetic, practical, and ideal for concurrent GPB and wheelchair use.[11]

Recently, noninvasive IPPV has been recognized as an effective alternative to tracheostomy IPPV and body ventilator use for nocturnal ventilatory support as well as for daytime aid.[14] Noninvasive IPPV is often introduced with the use of oximetry biofeedback. Mouthpiece IPPV with the mouthpiece held in the mouth or just adjacent to it is the most popular method of daytime ventilatory support (Fig. 3). Oximetry assists the patient with CAH in maintaining more normal daytime ventilation during strictly autonomous breathing as well as when supplementing tidal volumes with mouthpiece IPPV.[2,14] Patients should be instructed to keep their SaO_2 at or greater than 95% throughout the daytime hours and to supplement their breathing, if necessary, with periods of noninvasive IPPV.[12,13,18] The oximeter can gauge alveolar ventilation provided that supplemental oxygen is not used. Continuous SaO_2 monitoring is also especially useful during RTIs when continuous desaturation is a sign of atelectasis or pneumonia and sudden desaturation an indication of acute mucus plugging.

IPPV via nasal access is the most frequently preferred noninvasive IPPV method for nocturnal ventilatory support.[8,15,31,67,87] Custom interfaces may be used as in the treatment of sleep-disordered breathing (Fig. 1 and 2).[8,15,17] If nocturnal blood gas monitoring does not demonstrate sufficient normalization of ventilation with this method, then either mouthpiece

FIGURE 3. Forty-seven-year-old post-polio individual with no ventilator-free time except by glossopharyngeal breathing since onset at age 8. She was intubated and tracheostomized only once for a several-week period for a spinal derotation procedure. Otherwise, she has been using 24-hour mouthpiece IPPV since 1957 with the mouthpiece affixed adjacent to the sip-and-puff wheelchair controls.

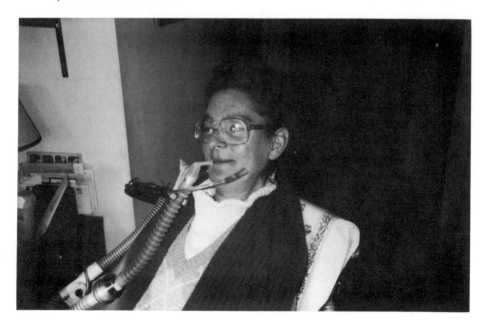

IPPV with a Bennett lipseal (Puritan-Bennett, Boulder, Colorado) or a custom-molded bite plate and lipseal should be tried.[13,14,18] A complete seal can be obtained even if one must plug the nose with cotton pledgets, cover it with a custom lipseal, and/or modify the mouthpiece or strap retention system for additional support.[14]

Ventilator volumes of 1,000 mL to greater than 2,000 ml may occasionally be necessary depending on the extent of ongoing insufflation air leakage. Pressure-cycled ventilators compensate at least partially for insufflation leakage.

For PVAIs living alone who are unable to manage a strap retention system, a strapless oral-nasal interface can be constructed.[17,70]

Thus, for all three methods, air can be delivered via comfortable, custom-molded interfaces. The use of nasal or mouthpiece IPPV with a capped tracheostomy tube is also an excellent alternative to ventilator weaning by tracheostomy IPPV in intermittent mandatory ventilation mode, pressure support ventilation, and progressive ventilator-free breathing/T-piece weaning and intermittent CPAP approaches.

Avoiding or eliminating a tracheostomy permits the patient to more readily learn GPB. GPB should be taught to those with less than 1,000 mL of VC and adequate oropharyngeal muscle strength for functional swallowing and speech.[12,35,36] GPB consists of use of the tongue and the pharyngeal muscles to add to a maximal inspiratory effort by projection of boluses of air past the vocal cords into the lungs. Effective GPB permits a patient to sustain ventilation for hours despite having little or no measurable VC (Fig. 4). It also normalizes speech production and provides deeper breaths for shouting and increasing PCEF. Progress with GPB should be monitored by regular measurement of the volume of air per gulp and the number of gulps per breath.

Although noninvasive IPPV methods are preferable to NPBVs or tracheostomy for long-term ventilatory support, NPBVs continue to be useful as temporary support for some patients during RTIs.[12,18] They can also be used during tracheostomy site closure,[9] for patients whose chronic aerophagia and abdominal distention are significantly exacerbated by noninvasive IPPV, and for the rare patient who simply prefers them to noninvasive IPPV.

In one study, 143 PVAIs with a mean VC of 734 ± 573 mL in the sitting position were mechanically ventilated by noninvasive methods.[10] Seventy-one patients were late-onset PVAIs beginning aid at age 41.9 ± 14.2 years (range, 9–78 years)—a mean of 29 ± 12.1 years (range, 3–59 years) post polio. These PVAIs benefited from ventilatory assistance a mean of 11.55 ± 9.1 years. Three of the 71 required only daytime ventilatory as-

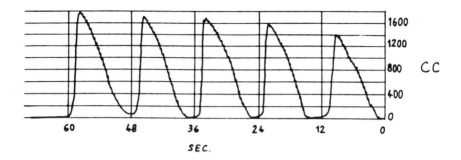

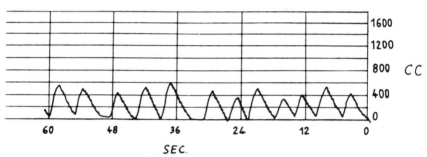

FIGURE 4. Top: Maximal GPB minute ventilation 8.39 lt, GPB inspirations average 1.67 lt, 20 gulps, 84 cc/gulp for each breath in a patient with a vital capacity of 0 cc. Bottom: Same patient regular GPB minute ventilation 4.76 lt/min, 12.5 breaths, average 8 gulps per breath, 47.5 cc/gulp performed over one minute period. (From Bach JR, et al: Glossopharyngeal breathing and non-invasive aids in the management of post-polio respiratory insufficiency. Birth Defects 23(4):99–113, 1987, with permission.)

sistance. Seventeen of the 71 used ventilatory aids overnight only. Ten others used them overnight and up to 8 hours during the daytime. The other 41 late-onset PVAIs progressed to require ventilatory assistance about 24 hours a day. All but 2 of these PVAIs required ventilatory assistance temporarily at onset of polio. The other 72 PVAIs were ventilator assisted from polio onset. They benefited from noninvasive aids for 37.5 ± 3.6 years.

Thirty-five of the 143 PVAIs had tracheostomies placed for management of acute medical or surgical conditions. Eleven PVAIs retained the tracheostomy for continued ventilatory assistance. Five of these 11 PVAIs died, all within 4 years of tracheostomy placement, from pulmonary disease associated with mucus plugging and/or substance abuse in four cases and cor pulmonale in the other case. The other 24 PVAIs had the tracheostomy sites closed, and they returned to noninvasive ventilatory support. Several patients had been tracheostomized as many as three times but each time returned to noninvasive support. Of the 24 PVAIs who have been ventilator assisted for 25.5 ± 13.7 years, only one has died thus far. Her death was associated with substance abuse.

The avoidance of tracheostomy in this group as a whole has permitted 59 of these PVAIs to master GPB sufficiently to use it for ventilator-free time. The 59 PVAIs with an average VC of 481 ml in the sitting position had an average GPmaxSBC of 2,133 ml. Their average ventilator-free time was increased by a mean of 2 hours by using GPB and was the only factor that permitted ventilator-free time for 24 PVAIs.

ASSISTED COUGHING

Because chest physical therapy techniques have not been shown to be effective in preventing or treating pneumonia and have not been shown to be more useful than effective coughing alone,[37,42,72] manually assisted coughing including the use of abdominal thrusts and mechanically assisted coughing should be used as necessary. Mechanically assisted coughing should be used when manual techniques are inadequate to generate 5 L/s of PCEF. This is often the case for patients with severe scoliosis or obesity. Mechanically assisted expulsion of airway secretions, which is both less labor-intensive and more effective, can be achieved with mechanical insufflation-exsufflation devices (Fig. 5) (Mechanical In-Exsufflator, J.H. Emerson Co., Cambridge, Massachusetts, or OEM Cof-flator Portable Cough Machine, Shampaine Industries, St. Louis, Missouri).[2,9,18,23,24,85] These devices provide optimal insufflation via an oral-nasal mask or mouthpiece—needed for PVAIs with less than 1,500 ml of VC—followed by a decrease in pressure of about 80 cm H_2O over a 0.2-sec period in order to create a forced exsufflation of 6–11 L/s. An abdominal thrust may be timed to the machine's exsufflation cycle to further increase PCEF. Such expiratory flows carry airway secretions into the mouth or mask. This can immediately increase VC, maximum pulmonary airflows, and SaO_2.[3,20] Assisted coughing may be necessary every 10–15 minutes around the clock during RTIs.[2,85]

Other mechanical approaches for eliminating secretions are being evaluated. Some act by applying rapidly oscillating pressure changes to the chest wall or directly to the airway. Such methods may be particularly useful in combination with postural drainage techniques for individuals with COPD for whom assisted coughing is unable to adequately overcome airway obstruction and for patients with severe bulbar involvement who as-

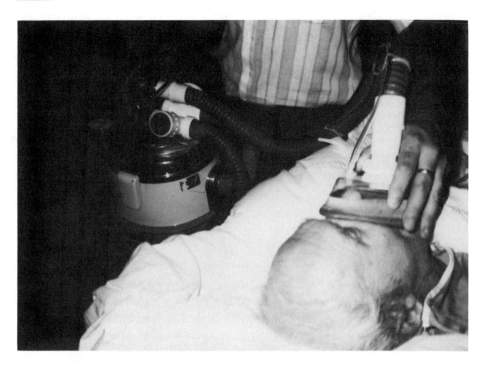

FIGURE 5. A Mechanical In-Exsufflator (Emerson Co., Cambridge, Massachusetts), which can be used alone or in conjunction with exsufflation timed abdominal thrusts to provide 6–11 L/s of peak cough expiratory flows and effective airway secretion elimination for patients with little or no ability of cough.

pirate oral secretions. For some patients, their use may also be beneficial prior to using manually or mechanically assisted coughing.

The application of high-frequency, chest wall compression to anesthetized dogs was found to maximize the tracheal mucus clearance rate at 11–15 Hz.[64] The Hayek oscillator can produce high-frequency oscillation to 160 Hz.[53] The variable I/E ratio permits variation in peak inspiratory and expiratory airway pressures (for example +3 to –6 cm H_2O), for a biased profile favoring mobilization of airway secretions.[47]

Intrapulmonary percussive ventilation has been reported to be more effective than chest percussion in the treatment of postoperative atelectasis and for secretion mobilization in general. The Percussionaire, Impulsator, and Spanker high-frequency percussive respirators (Percussionaire Corp., Sandpoint, Idaho) can deliver aerosolized medications while providing high-flow minibursts of air to the lungs at the rate of 2–7 Hz. In one study on 12 inpatients and 8 outpatients, sputum volume and FVC increased by 6% with regular use of intrapulmonary percussive ventilation. The majority of the patients felt that the treatments were helpful.[71] Jet ventilators are also being modified to provide biased pressure delivery profiles at wide frequency ranges to assist in airway secretion elimination.

TRACHEOSTOMY AND ITS INDICATIONS

Any patient without severe airway obstruction and with sufficient oropharyngeal muscle function to control saliva and to not require an indwelling gastrostomy tube for nutrition does not require an indwelling tracheostomy tube for ventilatory support or airway suctioning. Intubation and tracheostomy are associated with a high incidence of vocal cord paralysis and other complications that cause upper airway obstruction and instability and prevent eventual tracheostomy closure.

In the absence of intubation-associated upper airway complications, it is much easier to switch PVAIs from the use of body ventilators to the greatly preferred noninvasive IPPV techniques.[1] Bach et al. averted tracheostomy by converting more than 40 patients from suboptimal body ventilator use to noninvasive IPPV.[13,15] Intubation and tracheostomy can also be avoided in the intensive care setting.[9] Besides vocal cord paralysis, endotracheal intubation can also cause laryngitis, glottic edema, mucosal ulceration, laryngeal or tracheal stenosis, tracheal dilatation, tracheal-innominate artery fistula, atelectasis, and pulmonary infections.[21,59,60,76] Long-term tracheostomy is complicated by chronic bacterial colonization,[59,76] granulation tissue formation and bleeding, chronic mucus plugging, tracheal stenosis in 17–65% of patients, and many other less frequent but potentially serious complications, including accidental tracheostomy disconnection and respiratory arrest without possible resort to GPB.[39,46,75,80] Speech and swallowing are also hampered.[28]

In 1955, an International Consensus Symposium defined the indications for tracheostomy as the combination of respiratory insufficiency with swallowing insufficiency and disturbance in consciousness or vascular disturbances: "If a patient is going to be left a respirator cripple with a very low VC, a tracheotomy may be a great disadvantage. It is very difficult to get rid of a tracheotomy tube when the VC is only 500 or 600 cc and there is no power of coughing, whereas, as we all know, a patient who has been treated in a respirator from the first can survive and get out of all mechanical devices with a VC of that figure."[57] Although the indications for tracheostomy established in 1955 are equally appropriate today,[57] a tracheostomy is also indicated for patients with chronic ventilatory failure when PCEF by manually or mechanically assisted means cannot exceed 3 L/s because of irreversible airway obstruction, the MIC is less than 500 ml, there is a strong history of substance abuse, the patient is uncooperative, there are uncontrolled seizures, or there are orthopedic conditions that interfere with the use of masks for noninvasive IPPV.

OTHER REHABILITATION CONSIDERATIONS

Patient counseling should include an explanation of the therapeutic goals and how to attain them; the need to avoid unnecessary oxygen therapy, sedatives, heavy meals, extremes of temperature, humidity, excessive fatigue, exposure to respiratory tract pathogens, and obesity; the need for appropriate flu and bacterial vaccinations and early attention to maintaining alveolar ventilation and eliminating airway secretions during RTIs; how to prepare for any surgical procedures; and how to optimize daily functioning.

Basic rehabilitation methods include the use of lung expansion techniques by air stacking of mechanical insufflations[77] or GPB[12,35,36] to approach the MIC. This should be performed daily as the VC decreases to 50% of predicted normal. The earlier and more aggressively used, the better may be the ultimate effect on pulmonary compliance, alveolar surface tension, and the work of breathing. A positive pressure blower (Zephyr, Lifecare Inc., Lafayette, Colorado), IPPB machine, manual resuscitation, or portable ventilator is useful for delivering the mechanical insufflations.

Inspiratory muscle training has been shown to increase inspiratory muscle endurance for patients with progressive neuromuscular disease provided that the VC at onset of training is at least 30% of predicted normal.[40,69,74] These techniques may thus be of value for PPIs; it must be noted, however, that the greatest risk of complications occurs when the VC is 30% or less.[8]

PPIs require surgical intervention more frequently than the general population.[78] Preventive rehabilitation can prevent associated respiratory complications. A hospital of the patient's choice should be made aware of the patient's equipment and special needs. For the majority of hospitals that do not own portable ventilators, this might require advanced notice to the Risk and Claims services. Nursing and respiratory therapy in-services may be required.

The VC, PCEF, PCO_2, and SaO_2 are sensitive indicators of risk of postsurgical pulmonary complications. Except in the presence of CAH, it is unlikely that any patient with greater than 65% of predicted normal VC has greater risk of respiratory morbidity resulting from surgery and general anesthesia than does an individual with intact respiratory muscle function. The lower the VC below 60% and the PCEF below 5 L/s, the greater the likelihood of complications. Such patients or those with CAH of any etiology should be trained in receiving maximum insufflations with a portable ventilator by mouthpiece/lipseal and nasal IPPV in anticipation of postoperative ventilator weaning difficulties. Oximetry biofeedback may be useful. The PPI and his caregivers should also be introduced to both manually assisted and mechanically assisted coughing as described previously. Access to the latter is particularly important for patients who undergo abdominal surgery.[22,91] The use of Mechanical In-Exsufflators requires no abdominal muscle effort, and abdominal pressures are increased 70% less than during unassisted coughing.[25] Transient microatelectasis that might cause hypoxia can be reversed by frequent maximal insufflations and aggressive assisted coughing.

A patient who is fully alert following general anesthesia can be safely extubated whether or not capable of independently sustaining the ventilatory function. Immediately upon extubation, the patient should be ventilated by a mouthpiece or nasal mask and use nasal or lipseal IPPV during sleep with oximetry monitoring. The secretions stimulated by the intubation and anesthesia can be efficiently eliminated by assisted coughing methods. Pulmonary and laryngeal complications are averted by avoiding prolonged intubation. Likewise, during intercurrent RTIs, intubation, tracheostomy, and bronchoscopy almost always can be avoided by use of these noninvasive respiratory muscle aids.[6,14]

Since few centers have expertise in managing PVAIs who use noninvasive aids, it is important to contact a physician knowledgeable in their use for managing RTIs or when surgery is being considered. General anesthesia should be avoided in favor of local or regional anesthesia whenever possible and nonessential elective procedures avoided. Simple inhalation anesthetic techniques should be used whenever possible. Opioids and muscle relaxants should be used sparingly or avoided.[78] PVAIs should be returned to their ventilatory equipment as soon as alert postoperatively. Besides the differences in flow characteristics, the expiratory volume alarms of the usual hospital ventilators can make it impossible to use the 24-hour noninvasive ventilatory support techniques, which they may need and to which PPIs may already be accustomed. PVAIs with less than 2 hours of ventilator-free time should also have backup ventilators available.

ABBREVIATIONS AND GLOSSARY OF COMMON TERMS

Bi-Pap: Bilevel positive airway pressure: pressure assist ventilation in which inspiratory (IPAP) and expiratory (EPAP) assist pressures are individually set; used to splint open the hypopharynx during sleep for individuals with OSAS, to increase functional residual capacity, to decrease atelectasis, and to provide ventilatory assistance; the greater the IPAP/EPAP difference, the greater the inspiratory muscle (ventilatory) assist; can be used via a mouthpiece (with lipseal overnight) or nosepiece (most commonly a "CPAP mask").

CAH: Chronic alveolar hypoventilation: baseline blood carbon dioxide partial pressures chronically elevated (chronic hypercapnia).

COPD: Chronic obstructive pulmonary disease.

CPAP: Continuous positive airway pressure: same as Bi-PAP except that IPAP and EPAP pressures are equal; CPAP does not assist inspiratory muscle function and is, therefore, rarely useful for treating CAH.

EPAP: Expiratory positive airway pressure (*see* Bi-PAP).

GPB: Glossopharyngeal breathing: technique using pistoning movements of the tongue to create or increase tidal volumes; can be used to provide deep breaths to improve cough flows or increase voice volume and can be used to support alveolar ventilation for ventilatory supported individuals in the event of sudden ventilator failure.

GPmaxSBC: Glossopharyngeal maximum single breath capacity: the maximum depth glossopharyngeal breath; must be greater than VC.

IAPV: Intermittent abdominal pressure ventilator: a body ventilator used for inspiratory muscle (ventilatory) assistance with the subject in the sitting position.

Insufflation-exsufflation: Insufflation (mechanically assisted air entry into the lung) followed by sudden exsufflation (mechanical lung decompression) to create airflows for secretion elimination.

IPAP: Inspiratory positive airway pressure (*see* Bi-PAP).

IPPB: Intermittent positive pressure breathing: traditionally, pressure assist breathing used for medication, humidification, and deep breath delivery over short treatment periods via a mouthpiece.

IPPV: Intermittent positive pressure ventilation: essentially continuous pressure assist or volume assist IPPB used via oral, nasal, or oral-nasal interfaces for continuous ventilatory support.

IPV: Intrapulmonary percussive ventilation: the application of high-flow minibursts of air to the lungs at a rate of 2–7 Hz to enhance airway secretion elimination.

MIC: Maximum insufflation capacity: deepest insufflated breath that can be held with a closed glottis.

NPBV: Negative pressure body ventilator: inspiratory muscle (ventilatory) aids, which act by applying pressure to the body rather than directly to the airway.

OSAS: Obstructive sleep apnea syndrome: symptomatic individuals with greater than 10 apneas plus hypopneas per hour of sleep.

PCEF: Peak cough expiratory flow: may be greater than or, uncommonly, less than peak expiratory flows; may be assisted or unassisted.
PPIs: Post-paralytic poliomyelitis individuals.
PVAIS: Post-poliomyelitis ventilator-assisted individuals.
RTI: Respiratory tract infection.
SaO$_2$: Oxyhemoglobin saturation.
VC: Vital capacity.

REFERENCES

1. Bach JR: A comparison of long-term ventilatory support alternatives from the perspective of the patient and caregiver. Chest 104:1702, 1993.
2. Bach JR: Mechanical exsufflation, noninvasive ventilation and new strategies for pulmonary rehabilitation and sleep disordered breathing. Bull N Y Acad Med 68:321, 1992.
3. Bach JR: Mechanical insufflation-exsufflation: Comparison of peak expiratory flows with manually assisted and unassisted coughing techniques. Chest 104:1553, 1993.
4. Bach JR: Psychosocial aspects of home mechanical ventilation. In Kutscher AH (ed): The Ventilator: Psychosocial and Medical Aspects; Muscular Dystrophy, Amyotrophic Lateral Sclerosis, and Other Diseases. New York, Foundation of Thanatology, (in press).
5. Bach JR: Pulmonary Rehabilitation. In Mitchell CW, ed: Rehabilitation of the Aging and Older Patient. Baltimore, Williams & Wilkins, 1993, p. 263.
6. Bach JR: Pulmonary rehabilitation considerations for Duchenne muscular dystrophy: The prolongation of life by respiratory muscle aids. Crit Rev Phys Rehabil Med 3:239, 1992.
7. Bach, JR, Saporito, LR: Indications and criteria for decannulation and transition from invasive to noninvasive long-term ventilatory support. Respir Care 39:515, 1994.
8. Bach JR, Alba AS: Management of chronic alveolar hypoventilation by nasal ventilation. Chest 97:52, 1990.
9. Bach JR, Alba AS: Noninvasive options for ventilatory support of the traumatic high level quadriplegic. Chest 98:613, 1990.
10. Bach JR, Alba AS: Pulmonary dysfunction and sleep disordered breathing as postpolio sequelae: Evaluation and management. Orthopedics 14:1329, 1991.
11. Bach JR, Alba AS: Total ventilatory support by the intermittent abdominal pressure ventilator. Chest 99:630, 1991.
12. Bach JR, Alba AS, Bodofsky E, et al: Glossopharyngeal breathing and non-invasive aids in the management of post-polio respiratory insufficiency. Birth Defects 23:99, 1987.
13. Bach JR, Alba AS, Bohatiuk G, et al: Mouth intermittent positive pressure ventilation in the management of postpolio respiratory insufficiency. Chest 91:859, 1987.
14. Bach JR, Alba AS, Saporito LR: Intermittent positive pressure ventilation via the mouth as an alternative to tracheostomy for 257 ventilator users. Chest 103:174, 1993.
15. Bach JR, Alba AS, Shin D: Noninvasive airway pressure assisted ventilation in the management of respiratory insufficiency due to poliomyelitis. Am J Phys Med Rehabil 68:264, 1989.
16. Bach JR, Beltrame F: Alternative methods of ventilatory support. In Rothkopf MM, Askanazi J (eds): Home Intensive Care. Baltimore, Williams & Wilkins, 1992, p 173.

17. Bach JR, McDermott I: Strapless oral-nasal interfaces for positive pressure ventilation. Arch Phys Med Rehabil 71:908, 1990.

18. Bach JR, O'Brien J, Krotenberg R, Alba AS: Management of end stage respiratory failure in Duchenne muscular dystrophy. Muscle Nerve 10:177, 1987.

19. Bach JR, Penek J: Obstructive sleep apnea complicating negative pressure ventilatory support in patients with chronic paralytic/restrictive ventilatory dysfunction. Chest 99:1386, 1991.

20. Bach JR, Smith WH, Michaels J, et al: Airway secretion clearance by mechanical exsufflation for post-poliomyelitis ventilator assisted individuals. Arch Phys Med Rehabil 74:170, 1993.

21. Bain JA: Late complications of tracheostomy and prolonged endotracheal intubation. Int Anesthesiol Clin 10:225, 1972.

22. Barach AL, Beck GJ: Exsufflation with negative pressure: Physiologic and clinical studies in poliomyelitis, bronchial asthma, pulmonary emphysema and bronchiectasis. Arch Intern Med 93:825, 1954.

23. Barach AL, Beck GJ, Bickerman HA, et al: Physical methods simulating mechanisms of the human cough. J Appl Physiol 5:85, 1952.

24. Barach AL, Beck GJ, Smith RH: Mechanical production of expiratory flow rates surpassing the capacity of human coughing. Am J Med Sci 226:241, 1953.

25. Beck GJ, Scarrone LA: Physiological effects of exsufflation with negative pressure. Dis Chest 29:1, 1956.

26. Bergofsky EH: Cor pulmonale in the syndrome of alveolar hypoventilation. Prog Cardiovasc Dis 9:414, 1967.

27. Bickerman HA, Itkin S: Exsufflation with negative pressure. Arch Intern Med 93:698, 1954.

28. Bonanno P: Swallowing dysfunction after tracheostomy. Ann Surg 174:29, 1971.

29. Bonham PE, Currier GF, Orr WC, et al: The effect of a modified functional appliance on obstructive sleep apnea. Am J Orthod Dentofac Orthop 94:384, 1988.

30. Braun NMT, Arora NS, Rochester DF. Respiratory muscle and pulmonary function in polymyositis and other proximal myopathies. Thorax 38:616, 1983.

31. Carroll N, Branthwaite MA: Control of nocturnal hypoventilation by nasal intermittent positive pressure ventilation. Thorax 43:349, 1988.

32. Carskadon M, Dement W: Respiration during sleep in the aged human. J Gerontol 36:420, 1981.

33. Clark GT, Nakano M: Dental appliances for the treatment of obstructive sleep apnea. J Am Dent Assoc 118:611, 1989.

34. Curran FJ, Colbert AP: Ventilator management in Duchenne muscular dystrophy and postpoliomyelitis syndrome: Twelve years' experience. Arch Phys Med Rehabil 70:180, 1989.

35. Dail C, Rodgers M, Guess V, Adkins HV: Glossopharyngeal Breathing Manual. Downey, CA, Professional Staff Assoc., Rancho Los Amigos Hospital, 1979.

36. Dail CW, Affeldt JE: Glossopharyngeal Breathing [video], Los Angeles, Department of Visual Education, College of Medical Evangelists, 1954.

37. De Boeck C, Zinman R: Cough versus chest physiotherapy: A comparison of the acute effects on pulmonary function in patients with cystic fibrosis. Am Rev Respir Dis 129:182, 1984.

38. De Troyer A, Deisser P: The effects of intermittent positive pressure breathing on patients with respiratory muscle weakness. Am Rev Respir Dis 124:132, 1981.

39. Deutschman CS, Wilton P, Sinow J, et al: Paranasal sinusitis associated with nasotracheal intubation: A frequently unrecognized and treatable source of sepsis. Crit Care Med 14:111, 1986.

40. Dimarco AF, Kelling JS, DiMarco MS, et al: The effects of inspiratory resistive training on respiratory muscle function in patients with muscular dystrophy. Muscle Nerve 8:284, 1985.

41. Drinker PA, McKhann CF: The iron lung. JAMA 255:1476, 1986. 109. Eid N, Buchheit J, Neuling M, Phelps H: Chest physiotherapy in review. Resp Care 36:270, 1991.

42. Elam JO, Hemingway A, Gullickson G, Visscher MB: Impairment of pulmonary function in poliomyelitis: Oximetric studies in patients with the spinal and bulbar types. Arch Intern Med 81:649, 1948.

43. Enson Y, Giuntini C, Lewis ML, et al: The influence of hydrogen ion concentration and hypoxia on the pulmonary circulation. J Clin Invest 43:1146, 1964.

44. Estenne M, De Troyer A: The effects of tetraplegia on chest wall statics. Am Rev Respir Dis 134:121, 1986.

45. Fischer DA. Poliomyelitis: Late respiratory complications and management. Orthopedics 8:891, 1985.

46. Fishburn MJ, Marino RJ, Ditunno JF Jr: Atelectasis and pneumonia in acute spinal cord injury. Arch Phys Med Rehabil 71:197, 1990.

47. Freitag L, Long WM, Kim CS, Wanner A: Removal of excessive bronchial secretions by asymmetric high-frequency oscillations. J Appl Physiol 67:614, 1989.

48. George CF, Millar TW, Kryger MH: Identification and quantification of apneas by computer-based analysis of oxygen saturation. Am Rev Respir Dis 137:1238, 1988.

49. Goldstein RS, Molotiu N, Skrastins R, et al: Assisting ventilation in respiratory failure by negative pressure ventilation and by rocking bed. Chest 92:470, 1987.

50. Guilleminault C, Motta J: Sleep apnea syndrome as a long-term sequelae of poliomyelitis. In Guilleminault C (ed): Sleep Apnea Syndromes. New York, KROC Foundation, 1978, p 309.

51. Halstead LS, Wiechers DO, Rossi CD: Late effects of polio-myelitis: A national survey. In Halstead LS, Wiechers DO, eds: Late Effects of Poliomyelitis. Miami, Symposia Foundation, 1985, p 11.

52. Hamilton EA, Nichols PJR, Tait GBW: Late onset of respiratory insufficiency after poliomyelitis. Ann Phys Med 10:223, 1970.

53. Hayek Z, Ryan CA, Eyal F, et al: Comparison of high-frequency chest wall compression with conventional mechanical ventilation in cats. Crit Care Med 15:676, 1987.

54. He J, Kryger MH, Zorick FJ, et al: Mortality and apnea index in obstructive sleep apnea. Chest 94:9, 1988.

55. Hill R, Robbins AW, Messing R, Arora NS: Sleep apnea syndrome after poliomyelitis. Am Rev Respir Dis 127:129, 1983.

56. Historical Statistics of the United States: Colonial Times to 1970, Bicentennial Edition, Part 1. Washington, DC, U.S. Department of Commerce, Bureau of the Census, 1975, p 8, 77.

57. Hodes HL: Treatment of respiratory difficulty in poliomyelitis. In Poliomyelitis: Papers and Discussions Presented at the Third International Poliomyelitis Conference. Philadelphia, J.B. Lippincott, 1955, p 91.

58. Howard RS, Wiles CM, Spencer GT: The late sequelae of poliomyelitis. Q J Med 66:219, 1988.

59. Johanson WG, Pierce AK, Sanford JP, Thomas GD: Nosocomial respiratory infections with gram-negative bacilli: The significance of colonization of the respiratory tract. Ann Intern Med 77:701, 1972.

60. Johanson WG, Seidenfeld JJ, Gomez P, et al: Bacteriologic diagnosis of nosocomial pneumonia following prolonged mechanical ventilation. Am Rev Respir Dis 137:259, 1988.

61. Jubelt B, Cashman NR: Neurological manifestations of the post-polio syndrome. CRC Crit Rev Neurobiol 3:199, 1987.

62. Kaplan J, Fredrickson PA: Home pulse oximetry as a screening test for sleep-disordered breathing [abstract]. Chest 103(suppl)322S, 1993.

63. Katsantonis GP, Walsh JK, Schweitzer PK, Friedman WH: Further evaluation of uvulopalatopharyngoplasty in the treatment of obstructive sleep apnea syndrome. Otolaryngol Head Neck Surg 93:244, 1985.

64. King M, Phillips DM, Gross D, et al: Enhanced tracheal mucus clearance with high frequency chest wall compression. Am Rev Respir Dis 128:511, 1983.

65. Kinnear W, Petch M, Taylor G, Shneerson J: Assisted ventilation using cuirass respirators. Eur Respir J 1:198, 1988.

66. Lassen HCA: The epidemic of poliomyelitis in Copenhagen, 1952. Proc R Soc Med 47:67, 1953.

67. Leger P, Jennequin J, Gerard M, Robert D: Home positive pressure ventilation via nasal mask for patients with neuromuscular weakness or restrictive lung or chest-wall disease. Respir Care 34:73, 1989.

68. Lombard R Jr, Zwillich CW: Medical therapy of obstructive sleep apnea. Med Clin North Am 69:1317, 1985.

69. Martin AJ, Stern L, Yeates J, et al: Respiratory muscle training in Duchenne muscular dystrophy. Dev Med Child Neurol 28:314, 1986.

70. McDermott I, Bach JR, Parker C, Sortor S: Custom-fabricated interfaces for noninvasive intermittent positive pressure ventilation. Int J Prosthodont 2:224, 1989.

71. McInturff SL, Shaw LI, Hodgkin JE, et al: Intrapulmonary percussive ventilation in the treatment of COPD. Respir Care 30:885, 1985.

72. McMichan JC, Michel L, Westbrook PR: Pulmonary dysfunction following traumatic quadriplegia. JAMA 243:528, 1980.

73. Mier-Jedrzejowicz A, Brophy C, Green M: Respiratory muscle weakness during upper respiratory tract infections. Am Rev Respir Dis 138:5, 1988.

74. Milner-Brown HS, Miller RG: Muscle strengthening through high-resistance weight training in patients with neuromuscular disorders. Arch Phys Med Rehabil 69:14, 1988.

75. Moar JJ, Lello GE, Miller SD: Stomal sepsis and fatal haemorrhage following tracheostomy. Int J Oral Maxillofac Surg 15:339, 1986.

76. Niederman MS, Ferranti RD, Ziegler A, et al: Respiratory infection complicating long-term tracheostomy: The implication of persistent gram-negative tracheobronchial colonization. Chest 85:39, 1984.

77. O'Donohue W: Maximum volume IPPB for the management of pulmonary atelectasis. Chest 76:683, 1976.

78. Patrick JA, Meyer-Witting M, Reynolds F, Spencer GT: Peri-operative care in restrictive respiratory disease. Anaesthesia 45:390, 1990.

79. PetrénK, Ehrenberg L: Etudes cliniques sur la poliomyélite aigue. Nouv Inconog Salpétriére. 22:373, 546, 661, 1909.

80. Pingleton SK: Complications of acute respiratory failure. Am Rev Respir Dis 137:1463, 1988.

81. Plum F, Swanson AG: Abnormalities in central regulation of respiration in acute and convalescent poliomyelitis. Arch Neurol Psych 80:267, 1958.

82. Redline S, Tosteson T, Boucher MA, Millman RP: Measurement of sleep-related breathing disturbances in epidemiologic studies: Assessment of the validity and reproducibility of a portable monitoring device. Chest 100:1281–1286, 1991.

83. Riley RW, Powell NB, Guilleminault C, Mino-Murcia G: Maxillary, mandibular, and hyoid advancement: An alternative to tracheostomy in obstructive sleep apnea syndrome. Otolaryngol Head Neck Surg 94:584, 1986.

84. Smolley LA: Obstructive sleep apnea: Avoiding diagnostic pitfalls. J Respir Dis 11:547, 1990.

85. Sortor S, McKenzie M: Toward Independence: Assisted Cough [video]. Dallas, BioScience Communications of Dallas, 1986.

86. Splaingard ML, Frates RC, Jefferson LS, et al: Home negative pressure ventilation: Report of 20 years of experience in patients with neuromuscular disease. Arch Phys Med Rehabil 66:239, 1985.

87. Steljes DG, Kryger MH, Kirk BW, Millar TW: Sleep in postpolio syndrome. Chest 98:133, 1990.

88. Thawley SE: Surgical treatment of obstructive sleep apnea. Med Clin North Am 69:1337, 1985.

89. Waldhorn RE, Herrick TW, Nguyen MC, et al: Long-term compliance with nasal continuous positive airway pressure therapy of obstructive sleep apnea. Chest 97:33, 1990.

90. Williams AJ, Yu G, Santiago S, Stein M: Screening for sleep apnea using pulse oximetry and a clinical score. Chest 100:631, 1991.

91. Williams EK, Holaday DA: The use of exsufflation with negative pressure in postoperative patients. Am J Surg 90:637, 1955.

7

Respiratory Management in Late Post-Polio

JÖRGEN BORG, MD / JAN WEINBERG, MD

Respiratory disturbances during acute polio infection may be caused by lesions at different levels of the nervous system: the spinal cord produces respiratory muscle weakness, the cranial nerves produce bulbar muscle weakness, and the brainstem produces central drive failure.[40] Ten percent to 20% of patients with acute paralytic polio during the epidemics around 1950 in Western countries needed assisted ventilation.[26,29,32] The majority of surviving patients could be weaned off ventilators.[27,32]

In 1970, Hamilton et al. described patients with residuals after paralytic polio presenting with "a syndrome of late onset respiratory and circulatory insufficiency" characterized by "(a) increasing fatigue and depression, with decreasing memory, intellectual acuity, and capacity for intellectual work; (b) increasing dyspnea on exertion and increasing susceptibility to respiratory infection; (c) increasing sensitivity to cold, with cold extremities, peripheral cyanosis, and peripheral edema".[24] They claimed that the clinical syndrome might be recognized before there is a change in daytime blood gases and reported good effects of treatment with intermittent positive pressure ventilation. Since then, there have been several reports of late-onset post-polio respiratory insufficiency, including chronic hypoventilation,[2,27,31,38] nocturnal REM (rapid-eye-movement)–sleep-induced hypoxemia, and sleep apnea syndromes.[13,18,22,25] In a sur- **113** vey by Halstead et al., 42% of a late-post-polio population reported new breathing problems.[23]

Symptoms of late-post-polio respiratory problems might develop insidiously and are often related to nocturnal disturbances. Early recognition of symptoms and examination of noctural blood gases are important because adequate treatment can reduce symptoms, improve quality of life, and prevent severe cardiorespiratory complications including cor pulmonale and life-threatening CO_2 retention. Treatment has improved especially by the development of noninvasive techniques for intermittent positive pressure ventilation. The pathophysiology is multifactorial and might include declining respiratory muscle function. This chapter focuses on the early detection and treatment of late-onset post-polio respiratory disturbances and the possible role of diaphragmatic fatigue.

SYMPTOMS AND SIGNS

Symptoms of nocturnal respiratory disturbances include disturbed sleep, morning headache, daytime somnolence, and general fatigue.[2,24] These symptoms are probably caused by both sleep fragmentation and blood gas disturbances. Since symptoms are rather nonspecific, overlap with non-respiratory symptoms of the post-polio syndrome, and often develop insidiously, they might be neglected or misinterpreted. Often there is shortness of breath. While exercise-induced dyspnea might be pronounced in patients with significant restrictive pulmonary dysfunction but relatively well preserved extremity muscles, it will be minimal in patients with low demands due to the widespread muscle weakness that masks their low ventilatory capacity.

In advanced stages of diaphragmatic paresis, clinical examination might show paradoxical respiratory movements, with both inversion of the abdominal wall during the inspiration and use of accessory respiratory muscles during rest.

SLEEP RECORDINGS

Screening of nocturnal blood gas disturbances by whole-night monitoring of oxygen saturation and PCO_2 can be performed with noninvasive techniques applicable also in a patient's home, whereas a detailed analysis of breathing and sleep requires polygraphic recordings in a sleep laboratory.

Whole-night screening of oxygen saturation can be made by use of transcutaneous measurement through an ear or finger probe. Hypoxemia is characterized by permanent or periodic oxygen desaturation and/or apneas with episodic desaturations.[2,13,43] Whole-night screening of PCO_2 can be made either by analysis of end-tidal air, which parallels the arterial blood PCO_2 if there is no significant pulmonary disorder, or by transcutaneous measurement. Nocturnal hypoventilation is characterized by CO_2 retention of more than 13% during the night[37] or PCO_2 above 6.0 kPa (45 mm Hg).

Respiratory movement recordings support the interpretation of blood gas data. Recordings are made by use of either thoracical and abdominal electrodes or a static-charge-sensitive bed (SCSB).[46] SCSB yields information about periodic breathing; facilitates detection of upper airway obstruction, seen as a diamond-shaped breathing pattern; and permits an estimation of both movement-induced, false oxygen desaturations and the sleep time. Calculation of the oxygen desaturation index (ODI), which is the number of oxygen desaturations per sleep hour, corresponds to the apnea index.[47] An ODI below 4 is considered normal. Patients with an ODI of 4 or higher, a low basal oxygen saturation, or prolonged periods of desaturations should be referred for polysomnography (PSG) (according to the principles originally described by Gastaut.[19] PSG yields information on sleep time, on sleep stages, on movements of the chest and abdomen and on infrahyoidal muscle activity, as well as a semiquantification of airflow, which permits detection of apneas and hypopneas.

Bye et al. reported sleep-induced hypoxemia in 20 patients with respiratory muscle paresis due to different neuromuscular disorders including late post-polio.[13] They found that these patients typically maintained oxygen saturation during non-REM sleep but developed oxygen desaturation during REM sleep. The mean lowest oxygen saturation was 83% during non-REM and 60% during REM sleep. Mean daytime PO_2 was 8.9 kPa and mean daytime PCO_2 was 6.9 kPa. The awake blood gas levels were directly related to nocturnal oxygen desaturations. They suggested that the "extent of sleep induced hypoventilation is a key determinant of daytime $PaCO_2$ when they are awake."[13]

Steljes et al. reported polysomnographic results from 13 post-polio patients all having symptoms including increasing fatigue.[43] One group used rocking beds and one group had no respiratory aids. All but 3 patients had impaired sleep quality related to hypoventilation or apneas.

In our experience with polygraphic sleep recordings in late-post-polio patients presenting with symptoms indicating nocturnal respiratory disturbances, the predominant findings were REM-sleep-related periods of lower mean oxygen saturation levels and episodic hypopneic/apneic oxygen desaturation with arousals in accordance with the reports related above.[48]

PATHOPHYSIOLOGIC FACTORS

The risk of late-occurring hypoventilation in post-polio subjects is related to the degree of restrictive pulmonary dysfunction due to respiratory muscle weakness and/or kyphoscoliosis. Hypercapnia due to respiratory muscle weakness is usually seen only when the vital capacity is below 55% of the predicted.[12,13]

Late-onset hypoventilation has been observed in patients with residuals after respiratory muscle paresis both with and without need of assisted ventilation during acute paralytic polio. In a long-term follow-up of 209 patients, Howard et al. reported that 38% required assisted ventilation after a mean latent period of 33 years.[27] Of these, 45.5% did not require assisted ventilation during the acute period but were supposed to have had severe respiratory muscle weakness during the acute illness. Patients with late-onset need of assisted ventilation had vital capacities below 1.8 L.

In late-post-polio patients, restrictive pulmonary dysfunction might increase due to declining neuromuscular function and increasing thoracic deformities. Loss of vital capacity is related to respiratory muscle weakness and is more pronounced in a post-polio population compared to healthy subjects.[2,18] Patients with kyphoscoliosis have decreased chest wall compliance and decreased functional residual capacity (FRC). The lower FRC might reduce pulmonary oxygen, making a desaturation more pronounced for a given time of apnea or hypopnea.[17] The effect of ventilation-perfusion mismatch in scoliosis might also impair the respiratory function.[28]

In late post-polio, as in other neuromuscular disorders affecting respiratory muscles, chronic hypoventilation with severe CO_2 retention is probably preceded by intermittent nocturnal hypoxemia during REM sleep.[13] In patients with severe restrictive pulmonary dysfunction there is a fall in the vital capacity from the erect to the supine position.[13,37,38] Bye et al. reported a relation between the percentage fall of vital capacity from erect to the supine position and nocturnal hypoxemia as well as daytime blood gases.[13] Other factors contributing to nocturnal hypoventilation are reduced central drive of accessory respiratory muscles, reduced upper airway tonus, and reduced ventilatory responses to CO_2 and hypoxemia during REM sleep.[44] However, some patients seem to be able to use accessory muscles also during REM sleep.[45]

Obstruction of upper airways during sleep increases the workload on inspiratory muscles. Obesity and weak bulbar muscles might contribute. The coexistence of obstructive lung disease increases respiratory muscle work, and acute infection increases metabolic demands. Weak abdominal muscles might cause impaired drainage of the upper airways, thus predisposing to infections and atelectasis. Ambulatory patients might basically have larger metabolic demands with regard to extremity muscle activity compared to those confined to wheelchairs, which means increased risk for respiratory insufficiency.

DIAPHRAGMATIC FATIGUE

Respiratory muscles exhibit the same basic properties as other skeletal muscles including fatigability. Regarding the key role of the diaphragm in inspiratory capacity, knowledge about diaphragmatic fatigue is crucial to an understanding of respiratory failure in neuromuscular disorders including late post-polio. The various definitions of muscle fatigue reflect the complex mechanisms involved and the different methods used to describe those mechanisms. In a recent consensus report on respiratory muscle fatigue, it was suggested that muscle fatigue be defined as "a loss in the capacity for developing force and/or velocity of a muscle, resulting from muscle activity under load and which is reversible by rest" and that "fatigue precedes task failure, and thus, if it occurs clinically, it should precede the development of hypercapnia."[39]

The capacity of a muscle to develop force and velocity is related to different neuromuscular characteristics, including the muscle fiber properties. In the human diaphragm, type I and type II muscle fiber proportions are about equal; of the type II fibers there are about equal proportions of type A and B.[35] Although muscle fiber data from respiratory muscles in late post-polio are not available, some data from gait muscle studies, as described elsewhere in this book are of interest. Muscle biopsy studies of gait muscles have shown significant muscle fiber hypertrophy,[9,21] and an increased proportion of type 1 muscle fibers probably due to transformation of type II to type I muscle fibers in response to excessive use.[9] Isokinetic studies indicate that those fibers retain their type II contractile properties.[49] The hypertrophic fibers have a decreased number of capillaries per unit area and decreased metabolic enzyme content.[10,21] Even if these data do not permit any conclusions with regard to diaphragmatic function, they illustrate the significant changes of skeletal muscle fibers that might occur in response to new demands probably also in the diaphragm.

Even though muscle biopsy studies of the diaphragm are not possible in a living human there are methods to estimate the functional capacity of respiratory muscle including the diaphragm. Maximal inspiratory and expiratory mouth pressures have been used as a global estimate of respiratory muscle function. Phrenic nerve stimulation during maximal inspiratory efforts permits evaluation of central drive failure.[5] Calculation of the transdiaphragmatic pressure (Pdi) has been used to estimate diaphragmatic strength[6]. Pdi is defined as the difference between the abdominal (Pga) and the esophageal pressure (Pes). The maximal transdiaphragmatic pressure (Pdi max) is obtained by a maximal inspiratory effort against closed airways. The duty cycle of the diaphragm (Ti/Ttot) is calculated as the inspiratory time (Ti) relative to the length of the breathing cycle (Ttot). The tension time index (TTdi) is the product of the Pdi/Pdi max and Ti/Ttot and can be calculated for each breath.

Bellemare and Grassino found that in healthy subjects, breathing could be sustained more than 45 minutes when TTdi was at or below 0.15, and could be sustained less than 45 minutes when TTdi exceeded 0.15 and that the power spectrum of the diaphragmatic electromyogram (EMG) shifted toward lower frequencies at TTdi levels of 0.15.[6]

Using the same method, Sinderby et al studied five late-post-polio subjects using intermittent positive pressure ventilators.[41,42] Vital capacities ranged from 1.1 to 2.1 L (24–43% of the predicted). The center frequency of the diaphragmatic EMG signal (Cfdi) was used as an EMG index of localized diaphragmatic fatigue. All patients had elevated TTdi levels already at rest. During short-term arm or leg exercise, at levels corresponding to those that might occur in everyday life, TTdi increased to about 0.15 and exceeded that level in two. All but one patient showed a decrease in Cfdi. In summary, that study indicated a marked reduction in the force reserve at rest and a lower threshold to EMG fatigue than observed in healthy subjects.[6] All patients in the study had been subjected to polygraphic sleep and blood gas recordings. Two were normal and the others showed sleep-related respiratory disturbances.

MONITORING OF AT-RISK PATIENTS

Clinical symptoms and signs of respiratory disturbances should be evaluated by pulmonary function tests and nocturnal examination. All patients with symptoms indicating nocturnal respiratory disturbances should be examined by a screening of nocturnal blood gases including whole-night monitoring of oxygen saturation and CO_2 tension. If normal, the screening should be repeated if symptoms progress. If there are signs of nocturnal blood gas disturbances, a polygraphic sleep recording is recommended in order to characterize the respiratory disturbances, evaluate sleep quality, and design the treatment.

All patients with a vital capacity of less than 55% should be examined by means of nocturnal blood gas recordings in order to detect subclinical respiratory disturbances and get a baseline for further controls. If there are no signs of nocturnal blood gas disturbances, we recommend that the nocturnal blood gas screen be performed either if symptoms appear or, otherwise, annually.

PREVENTION AND TREATMENT

Prevention of respiratory insufficiency includes physiotherapy to improve chest wall and pulmonary compliance and mucus drainage. Physiotherapy might include the exercise training of nonaffected accessory muscles. To our knowledge there are no reports of long-term follow-up studies on the exercise training of weak respiratory muscles in late post-polio.

Physiotherapy might also include the teaching of frog breathing. Bach and Alba recommend this for patients with a vital capacity less than 1000 mL and with adequate oropharyngeal muscle strength.[2] In addition, dietary factors and weight control should be considered.

ASSISTED VENTILATION

Assisted ventilation should be considered in patients with significant restrictive pulmonary dysfunction and nocturnal examination showing sleep-induced hypoxemia or CO_2 retention. Further studies are needed to determine if assisted ventilation should be introduced in order to reduce diaphragmatic fatigue[39] before significant blood gas changes occur.

There are now several reports of intermittent positive pressure ventilation (IPPV) using noninvasive oral or nasal access.[3,4,14,16,30,33] IPPV via nasal access is often the better alternative. Oral access might be better in patients with air leakage through the mouth due to weak oral muscles, but it might cause problems due to dehydration and the air leakage. Methods based on application of negative pressure, such as the iron lung and the cuirass, are less comfortable and less effective and might even be hazardous due to induction of upper airway obstruction.[34] Tracheostomy is effective but more disabling and thus not the method of first choice when only nighttime ventilation is needed, but it should be considered if noninvasive methods are not sufficient.[2]

Several portable volume- or pressure-conducted ventilators are available. Individual preferences differ due to their different airflow characteristics and due to other factors such as the weight and noise level of the equipment. Connection of the ventilator by nasal access can be by way of commercially available preformed masks or the SEFAM mask molded by a commercially available kit (from Lifecare, Inc.). When there are problems due to air leakage, discomfort, or skin pressure, custom-fabricated nasal masks might be an alternative. Recently, we evaluated a new nasal mask made by visible-light-curing acrylic (Figs. 1 and 2).

Introduction of a respiratory aid requires adequate education of the patient and, when relevant, the family and the nursing staff. Continuous support by a specialized team that includes an experienced respiratory physiotherapist and a technician is necessary. Regular treatment evaluation is important and should include nocturnal blood gas screening during ventilator use. In the long run there might be a need for adjustment of the ventilator settings as well as of the nasal mask.

The beneficial effects of nocturnal assisted ventilation manifested as reduced symptoms in response to normalized blood gases and sleep pattern might also be related to restored chemoreceptor settings, improved tissue compliance, and improved respiratory muscle function. The possible role

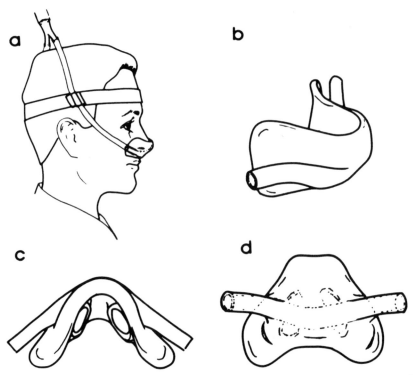

FIGURE 1. Nasal mask for nocturnal ventilation: (a) connected, (b) lateral view, (c) dorsal view, (d) frontal view. (From Klefbeck B, Remmer L, Weinberg J, Borg J: A new nasal mask for home ventilation in chronic neuromuscular disorders. Scand J Rehabil Med 25:7–9, 1993, with permission.)

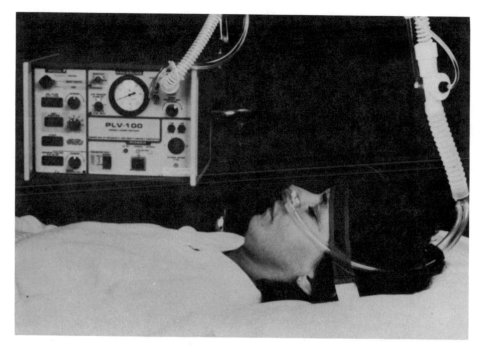

FIGURE 2. The patient connected to a PLV 100. (From Klefbeck B, Remmer L, Weinberg J, Borg J: A new nasal mask for home ventilation in chronic neuromuscular disorders. Scand J Rehabil Med 25:7–9, 1993, with permission.)

of diaphragmatic fatigue is indicated by the beneficial effects on respiratory muscle strength and endurance as reported after assisted ventilation.[17,20,36]

Patients without restrictive pulmonary dysfunction and signs of sleep apnea should be treated according to the same principles as usual in this condition.[44]

SUMMARY

Late-post-polio patients are at risk for the insidious development of nocturnal respiratory disturbances. Early symptoms are often nonspecific, so diagnosis is based on nocturnal blood gas recordings. In patients with significant restrictive pulmonary dysfunction and signs of nocturnal hypoxemia or hypercapnia, assisted ventilation by noninvasive techniques should be considered. Further studies are needed to determine whether this treatment should be introduced in order to reduce diaphragmatic fatigue before significant blood gas disturbances arise.

REFERENCES

1. Bach JR, Alba AS: Management of chronic alveolar hypoventilation in by nasal ventilation. Chest 97:52–57, 1990.

2. Bach JR, Alba AS: Pulmonary dysfunction and sleep disordered breathing as postpolio sequelae: Evaluation and management. Orthopedics 14:1329–1337, 1991.

3. Bach JR, Alba AS, Mosher R, Delaubier A: Intermittent postive pressure ventilation via nasa access in the management of respiratory insufficiency. Thorax 92:168–170, 1987.

4. Bach JR, Alba AS, Shin D: Noninvasive airway pressure assisted ventilation in the management of respiratory insufficiency due to poliomyelitis. Am J Phys Med Rehabil 68:264–271, 1989.

5. Bellemare F, Bigland Ritchie B: Central components of diaphragamtic fatigue assessed by phrenic nerve stimulation. J Appl Physiol 62:1307–1316, 1987.

6. Bellemare F, Grassino A: Effects of pressure and timing of contraction on human diaphragm fatigue. J. Appl. Physiol Respir Environ Exerc Physiol 53:1190–1195, 1982.

7. Bellemare F, Grassino A: Evaluation of human diaphragm fatigue. J Appl Physiol Environ Exerc Physiol 53:1196–1206, 1982.

8. Bergofsky H: Respiratory failure in disorders in the thoracic cage. Am Rev Respir Dis 119:6432–669, 1979.

9. Borg K, Borg J, Edström L, Grimby L: Effects of excessive use of remaining muscle fibers in prior polio and LV root lesion. Muscle Nerve 11:1219–1148, 1988.

10. Borg K, Henriksson J: Prior poliomyelitis-reduced capillary supply and metabolic enzyme content in hypertrophic slow-twitch (type I) muscle fibres. J Neurol Neurosurg Psychiatry 54:236–240, 1991.

11. Borg J, Weinberg J, Klefbeck B: When is assisted ventilation indicated in neuromuscular disease [abstract]? J Neurol Sci 98:342, 1990.

12. Braun N, Arora N, Rochester D: Respiratory muscle and pulmonary function in polymyositis and other proximal myopathies. Thorax 38:616–623, 1983.

13. Bye PTB, Ellis ER, Issa FG, Donnelly PM, Sullivan CE: Respiratory failure and sleep in neuromuscular disease. Thorax 45:241–247, 1990.

14. Carrol N, Branthwaite M: Intermittent positive pressure ventilation by nasal mask: technique and applications. Intens Care Med 14:115–117, 1988.

15. Ellis E, Bye P, Bruderer J, Sullivan C: Treatment of respiratory failure during sleep in patients with neuromuscular disease: Positive pressure ventilation through a nose mask. Am Rev Respir Dis 135:148–152, 1987.

16. Ellis E, Grunstein R, Shu-Chan, et al: Noninvasive ventilatory support during sleep improves respiratory failure in kyphoscoliosis. Chest 94:811–815, 1988.

17. Findley L, Ries A, Tisi G, Wagner P: Hypoxemia during apnea in normal subjects: Mechanisms and impact of lung volume. J Appl Physiol Respir Environ Exerc Physiol 55:1777–1783, 1983.

18. Fischer DA: Poliomyelitis: Late respiratory complications and maagement. Orthopedics 8:891–894, 1985.

19. Gastaut H, Tassinari, Duron B: Etude polygraphique des manifestations episodiques (hypniques et respiratoires) du syndrome de Pickwick. Rev Neurol 112:569–579, 1965.

20. Goldstein R, De Rosie J, Avendano M, Dolmage T: Influence of noninvsive positive pressure ventilation on inspiratory muscles. Chest 99:408–415, 1991.

21. Grimby G, Einarsson G, Hedberg M, Aniansson A: Muscle adaptive changes in post-polio subjects. Scand J Rehabil Med 21:19–26, 1989.

22. Guilleminault C, Motta J: Sleep apnea syndrome as a long term sequelae of poliomyelitis. In Guilleminault C, Dement WC, eds: Sleep Apnea Syndromes. New York, Alan R. Liss, 1978, pp 309–315.

23. Halstead LS, Wiechers DO, Rossi CD: Late effects of poliomyelitis: A national survey. In Halstead LS, Wiechers DO (eds): Late Effects of Poliomyelitis. Miami, Symposia Foundation, 1985.

24. Hamilton E, Nichols P, Tait G: Late onset respiratory insufficiency after poliomyelitis. Ann Phys Med 10:223–229, 1970.

25. Hill R, Robbins AW, Messing R, Arora NS: Sleep apnea syndrome after poliomyelitis. Am Rev Resprir Dis 127:129–131, 1983.

26. Hodes HL: Treatment of respiratory difficulty in poliomyelitis. In Papers and Discussions Presented at the Third International Poliomyelitis Conference. Philadelphia, J.B. Lippincott, 1955, pp 91–113.

27. Howard RS, Wiles CM, Spencer GT: The late sequelae of poliomyelitis. Q J Med 66(251):219–232, 1988.

28. Kafer ER: Idiopathic scoliosis: Gas exchange and the age dependence of arterial blood gases. J Clin Invest 58:825–833, 1976.

29. Kaufert PL, Kaufert JM: Methodological and conceptual issues in measuring the long term impact of disability: The experience of poliomyelitis patients in Manitoba. Soc Sci Med 19:609–618, 1984.

30. Klefbeck B, Remmer L, Weinberg J, Borg J: A new nasal mask for home ventilation in chronic neuromuscular disorders. Scand J Rehabil Med 25:7–9, 1993.

31. Lane DJ, Hazleman B, Nichols PRJ: Late onset respiratory failure in patients with previous poliomyelitis. Q J Med 172:551–568, 1974.

32. Lassen HCA: The epidemic of poliomyelitis in Copenhagen, 1952. Proc R Soc Med 47:6–71, 1953.

33. Leger P, Jennequin M, Gerard M, et al: Home positive pressure ventilation via nasal mask for patients with neuromusculoskeletal disorders. Eur Respir J 2(Suppl 7):640–645, 1989.

34. Levy R, Bradley D, Newman S, et al: Negative pressure ventilation: Effects on ventilation during sleep in normal subjects. Chest 95:95–99, 1989.

35. Liebermann DA, Faulkner JA, Craig AB, Maxwell LC: Performance and histochemical composition of guinea pig and human diaphragm. J Appl Physiol 34:233–237, 1973.

36. Marino W, Braun N: Reversal of the clinical sequele of the respiratory muscle fatigue by intermittent mechanical ventilation. Am Rev Respir Dis 125(2A):1982.

37. Midgren B: Continuous non-invasive assessment of blood gases during sleep [thesis]. Lund, University Hospital Lund, 1987.

38. Newsom Davis J, Goldman M, Loh L, Casson M: Diaphragm function and alveolar hypoventilation. Q J Med 45(177):87–100, 1976.

39. NHLBI Workshop Summary: Fatigue. Am Rev Respir Dis 142:474–480, 1990.

40. Plum F, Swanson AG: Abnormalities in central regulation of respiration in acute and convalescent poliomyelitis. Arch Neurol Psych 80:267–285, 1958.

41. Sinderby C, Weinberg J, Lindström L, Grassino A: Respiratory muscle force reserve in patients with chronic cervical cord injuries and in patients with prior polio infection [thesis]. Gothenburg, University of Gothenburg, 1991.

42. Sinderby C, Weinberg J, Sullivan L, et al: Respiratory muscle function at rest and exercise in patients with cervical cord injuries and in patients with prior polio infection [thesis]. Gothenburg, University of Gothenburg, 1991.

43. Steljes D, Kryger M, Kirk B, Millar T: Sleep in postpolio syndrome. Chest 98:133–140, 1990.

44. Sullivan C, Issa E, Bruderer J, et al: Treatment of cardiorespiratory disturbances during sleep. Interdisc Topics Geront 22:47–67, 1987.

45. Svanborg E, Borg J, Weinberg J: Sleep and respiration in chronic neuromuscular disorders [abstract]. J Neurol Sci 98:342, 1990.

46. Svanborg E, Larsson H, Carlsson-Nordlander B, Pirskanen R: A limited diagnostic investigation for obstructive sleep apnea syndrome: Oximetry and static charge sensitive bed. Chest 98:1341–1345, 1990.

47. Svanborg E, Larsson H, Nordlander B, Pirskanen R: Static charge sensitive bed and oximetry recordings in the study of obstructive sleep apnea syndrome. In Guilleminault C, Partinen M, eds: Obstructive Sleep Apnea Syndrome: Clinical Research and Treatment. New York, Raven Press, 1990, pp 195–207.

48. Svanborg E, Weinberg J, Borg J: Abnormalities of respiration and sleep in neuromuscular disorders. In manuscript.

49. Tollbäck A, Knutsson, E, Borg J, et al: Torque-velocity relation and muscle fibre characteristics of foot dorsiflexors after long-term overuse of residual muscle fibres due to prior polio or L5 root lesion. Scand J Rehabil Med 24:151–156, 1992.

8

Long-Term Effects of Post-Polio on Oral-Motor and Swallowing Function

BARBARA C. SONIES, PhD

Some persons who suffered an acute attack of poliomyelitis well over 30 years ago are experiencing new symptoms of muscle weakness, fatigue, and varying degrees of pain. It had been assumed by many that these new symptoms were unrelated to their original episode.[3] Some individuals were told by their physician that they were having a psychological overreaction and should seek counseling. For others, the symptoms suggested diagnosis of a new neurological disorder such as amyotrophic lateral sclerosis and led to feelings of fear, anxiety, and frustration.[18]

Various opinions have been expressed to explain the etiology of these new symptoms in those who survived the polio epidemic of the 1950s. One hypothesis was that the poliovirus was reactivated. Another presumed that the condition was actually a form of aging that was exacerbated by the original loss of motor neurons during the polio infection or that the anterior horn cells of the spinal cord had become overloaded.[27] Another suggested that some of the cells in the spinal cord had survived in a damaged form and could not function adequately.[8–13] More recently, the thinking on the post-polio syndrome indicates that the condition may be the result of overuse of the remaining previously healthy motor neurons, causing slow degeneration of the terminals of individual nerve axons.[8–11,16]

Regardless of the specific reason for new symptoms, it has become evident that in many individuals, the oropharyngeal musculature is affected in a manner similar to that of the proximal and distal muscles. Therefore, in addition to the emergence of changes in gait, balance, trunk, body control, and hand motion, new speech and swallowing deficits may appear in persons who had polio. Because these oropharyngeal deficits imply subclinical dysfunction of the bulbar muscles that may exacerbate over time, it is especially important that individuals develop increased awareness of dysphagia and its evolution. Whereas the progression of most symptoms in post-polio is disabling, the complications associated with difficulty in swallowing, such as aspiration pneumonia, are serious and can often be life threatening. This chapter reviews some of the controversies suggested by previous studies and the areas of common agreement regarding the prevalence, evolution, diagnosis, and treatment of speech, voice, and swallowing disorders.

HISTORICAL PERSPECTIVES

Investigators have suggested a variety of names for this condition, which could affect half of the original 1.63 million U.S. polio survivors, including post-polio syndrome, post-polio progressive muscular atrophy, the late affects of polio, and post-polio sequelae.[3] Most agree that post-polio progressive muscular atrophy (PPMA) is most appropriate.[5,6,10,13,14] According to Halstead, there are five criteria that must exist in order for this condition to be fit into a proper diagnosis of PPMA.[14] The criteria are (1) confirmed previous history with electromyograhic (EMG) findings, (2) a specific EMG pattern, (3) a stable period of neurological recovery of more than 20 years, (4) gradual or abrupt appearance of new symptoms in previously affected or unaffected muscles that may be coupled with other health symptoms, and (5) exclusion of other neurologic conditions that could cause similar deficits.[14]

Dalakas suggests there are several factors that must be present in order for post-polio syndrome to be considered: (1) severe acute paralytic disease, (2) older age at onset of acute illness, and (3) severe residual disability.[8] He also suggests that residual deficits must consist of asymmetric weakness, atrophy of one or more limbs, areflexia, normal sensation, and electrophysiologic signs of denervation.[9–11]

Insidious onset, fatigue, loss of stamina, and joint and muscle pains have also been included in the description of the late-emerging condition.[18]

Most agree that the more severe the original condition, the greater the likelihood that later-developing symptoms will occur. Although there has been some controversy as to whether persons without early bulbar symptoms would have new signs of speech and swallowing dysfunction, one study suggested that new symptoms may not always correspond to the original symptoms and that reporters may be unaware of new symptoms until the symptoms become moderate in nature.[24] However, since normal aging does not cause decremental changes in the processes of speech and swallowing, any new signs of dysfunction would most likely be due to a neuromuscular change and thus merit special attention.[21,22]

PREVALENCE OF OROPHARYNGEAL SYMPTOMS

Fewer patients report oropharyngeal symptoms such as breathing and swallowing difficulty than they do problems with gait or activities of daily living.[14] In our experience in evaluating post-polio patients referred to the National Institutes of Health, we found that many are unaware of having any difficulty swallowing because they have learned to compensate for mild problems in transporting food or have accepted indigestion as a common mealtime sequelae.

Approximately 300,000 in the United States survived the 1940s and 1950s polio epidemics. Early estimates indicate that between 20% and 25% of survivors, (upwards of 75,000) will experience late effects (NINCDS:NIH:HHS Survey). Other more recent studies have found new symptoms occurring in 28.5–60% of survivors.[17,28] Although slow and insidious, it has been estimated that progression of symptoms occurs at a steady rate, varying from approximations of 1% to 9% per year.[1,12,28]

No large-scale survey has been conducted on the long-term effects of the post-polio syndrome on swallowing, but several studies have looked at small but representative population samples and have found consistent reports of dysphagia in the majority of patients who return for study. Since the discovery of the polio vaccine, recent yearly incidence of new cases of polio is very small, and any reports of dysphagia would be found only in those patients whose symptoms had resulted from the original illness.

Twenty patients were studied for a 2-year period at the University of Michigan's Post-Polio Clinics. Ten of the clinic's patients had difficult swallowing during their original attack of polio. Regardless of the original problem, all of the subjects began to experience symptoms of dysphagia from 17 to 43 years after their acute episode.[20] A few of the patients demonstrated speech resonance or respiratory/phonatory changes and became hoarse or had difficulty chewing or swallowing when fatigued. A large number of patients had oral motor weakness and an abnormal laryngeal examination.

In a 1953 study of 27 patients who had originally had pharyngeal weakness, Bosma found that the majority remained with weak pharyngeal constrictor muscles and palatal abnormalities at follow-up.[2]

Coelho and Ferranti found an 18% incidence of dysphagia in 220 polio survivors who responded to a swallowing function questionnaire.[7] Although their patients' symptoms ranged in severity, none of their patients aspirated during the examination. The researchers found that 17 of 20 patients with dysphagia had decreased breathing capacity; however, evidence of one deficit did not predict the other. The authors cautioned that their estimates were most likely conservative because individuals (screened by mail) who were not able to recall whether they had problems were not included in the study sample.

Using cinefluorography, Jones et al. evaluated 20 patients with a remote history of post-polio and found that all but one exhibited some degree of pharyngeal abnormality as well as other structural problems that had contributed to dysphagia.[15] Similar findings were noted by Buchholz in a study of 13 persons with post-polio and complaints of dysphagia.[4] Nine of these individuals had been originally diagnosed with bulbar symptoms, which would cause oropharyngeal impairment.

Sonies and Dalakas studied 32 patients chosen at random from a cohort of 72 patients with a diagnosis of PPMA.[23,24] Two patients had dysphagia as their dominant symptom. Despite the finding that 24 had had involvement of the bulbar muscles during their original illness, only 14 of the 32 patients reported being aware of symptoms of oropharyngeal dysphagia at the time of the study. Of the 24 patients reporting new swallowing difficulties, 18 had had a previous diagnosis of bulbar involvement. Of the 20 patients with nonbulbar type poliomyelitis at original diagnosis, five presented with new swallowing difficulty. This study suggested that regardless of whether or not the original type of poliomyelitis was bulbar of spinal, new swallowing symptoms may emerge as late effects. It also suggested that symptoms of dysphagia, ranging from mild to moderate, can be found in individuals regardless of whether or not the individual is aware of having any symptoms.

THE OROPHARYNGEAL SYSTEM

The oropharyngeal system is composed of the anatomical and neuromuscular structures and sensory end organs of the face, mouth, pharynx, larynx, esophagus, and lungs. These structures are innervated by cranial nerves V (trigeminal), VII (facial), IX (glossopharyngeal), X (vagal), and XII (hypoglossal). Sensory and motor control of respiration, phonation, taste, smell, speech, and deglutition is regulated by these cranial nerves.[21] Their respective cranial nerve nuclei, located in the brain stem (pons and medulla), are often referred to as the bulbar system. If these nuclei had been affected by the original illness, the individual would have been diagnosed with bulbar poliomyelitis. The original symptoms of those with bulbar poliomyelitis would have included one or more of the following signs of abnormality in the oropharyngeal system: dysarthria, dysphagia, aphonia, dysfluency, and breathing impairment. Although this chapter does not provide an in-depth discussion of impairment, a short description of the common findings of oropharyngeal system dysfunction follows.

SPEECH AND VOICE

The major speech change found in polio survivors is increased nasal resonance. This hypernasality is due to insufficient contact of the soft palate with the posterior pharyngeal wall, allowing air escape into the nasopharynx during speaking. The palate may be asymmetric or hemiparetic, or the muscles of the hypopharynx may be weakened. The effects of fatigue on the hyolaryngeal musculature coupled with weakness of the respiratory muscles often cause increased hoarseness, lowered pitch or volume, or loss of voice.[20,23] Sonies and Dalakas found that patients who were aware of having symptoms of dysphagia had more severe deficits in voice quality than those who were asymptomatic.[23] However, they did not find significant differences between the polio groups or between normal controls and post-polio patients on speech articulation or fluency. Although a few survivors have been described as having an articulatory impairment, this is not typical of post-polio and may have been coincidental rather than disease related (Table 1).

RESPIRATORY/PHONATORY CHANGES

Pulmonary changes caused by previously weak muscles of the diaphragm, ribs, or abdomen can produce shallow or irregular breathing, shortness of breath, or apnea. It is likely that affected individuals may have been able to compensate for minimal respiratory dysfunction for many years and then experienced rapid failure when these compensations became insufficient to maintain adequate respiratory support. Once the ability to maintain adequate respiration is impaired, speech and swallowing can become dysfunctional. Because speech depends on adequate breath support, respiratory deficiency causes impaired phonation with decreased volume and

TABLE 1. Major Speech and Voice Complaints in Post-Polio Patients

Hypernasality

Intermittent aphonia

Reduced volume

Hoarseness

improper phrasing. Swallowing can be viewed as reciprocal to breathing; breathing ceases at the moment the airway is protected for bolus passage through the pharynx. In the case of swallowing, incoordination of respiration/deglutition may result in aspiration and the serious complications of aspiration pneumonia.

ORAL SENSORIMOTOR FUNCTION

Results of detailed oral sensorimotor examinations have been reported in two studies of post-polio. Silbergleit et al. found unilateral weakness of the tongue or palate in 80% and laryngeal abnormalities in 57% of their patients.[20] Sonies and Dalakas used an oral motor index with ten categories of function to evaluate their subjects.[23] They compared symptomatic to asymptomatic patients on the following: oral structure: symmetry and volitional and reflexive movement of the tongue, lips, jaw, and palate: tongue and lip strength; swallowing ability; fluency; and oral diadochokinesis. A rating score of 1–4 (normal, mild, moderate, severe) was assigned to each category based on a 52-item, cranial nerve-based examination. Regardless of whether patients were symptomatic or asymptomatic, signs of mild to moderate abnormalities in oral motor function were found in all but one of the 32 patients. Both groups demonstrated tongue, lip, and jaw weakness and slowed or abnormal tongue, jaw, or palatal movements with slowed oral diadochokinesia. However, the deficits found in the symptomatic patients were significantly greater than those in the asymptomatic groups in all of the categories.

SWALLOWING

A clinical dysphagia evaluation, mealtime observation, and a questionnaire to determine patient's level of subjective awareness should be completed to adequately assess swallowing. Once the implications of those clinical examinations have been analyzed, instrumental diagnostic procedures should be administered to obtain an objective record of swallowing (i.e., videofluoroscopy, ultrasound).

CLINICAL EVALUATION OF DYSPHAGIA

This procedure consists of a complete oral sensorimotor examination, including an inventory of medications, allergies, and sensory changes; a medical history; description of the evolution and changes in symptoms, salivation, and eating habits. The examination will need to focus on whether the individual has weak facial or oral muscles or orofacial asymmetry or paresis and whether there are indications that bolus preparation and transport are impaired.[26] The strength and range of motion of the oral musculature should be assessed along with oral reflexes and dentition. The individual should be observed while eating to determine if drooling, choking, or coughing accompanies meals or if the patient avoids or rejects a particular type of food. It should be determined if pocketing of food in the buccal sulci or if residue on the tongue or teeth is present after several swallows. Any delays in eating and any unusual postures or positions should be noted. The most significant outcome of this portion of the examination is the determination of whether the bolus is being transported in the correct manner from the mouth through the pharynx.

Changes in voice quality such as harshness or gurgling sounds are indicative of residue on the vocal folds and a signal of later laryngeal penetration and possible aspiration. The strength of the cough and whether the throat can be cleared are important signals of ability to protect the airway from entry of harmful food material. Aspiration and silent aspiration occur most frequently in individuals who are unable to use the cough to clear the airway.

MEALTIME OBSERVATIONS

Whenever possible, the dysphagia diagnostician should attempt to watch the person ingest a typical meal. A family member can also be given instructions regarding the components of the observation. In addition, the information can be gathered in written form or from interview. This observation can provide the invaluable insights needed to develop treatment plans and it can be immediately reinforcing to the person with a swallowing disability. As was stressed in the clinical examination, the mealtime observation should be used to substantiate whether the individual is a safe oral feeder and whether modifications are needed to ensure mealtime safety.

SWALLOWING QUESTIONNAIRE

In order to determine whether the patient is aware of dysphagia, the diagnostician should have each individual complete a self-assessment questionnaire.[25] We use an 18-item screening tool instructing the patient to indicate whether a set of symptoms is present. We then administer another self-rating scale on which the individual indicates, using a scale of 1–4, the severity (normal, mild, moderate, severe) or occurrence (never, sometimes, often, always) of a particular set of behaviors based on the more general screening (Appendix A). Some of the more common complaints elicited from post-polio patients by the questionnaire include intermittent choking on foods, pills sticking in the throat, difficulty swallowing pills, food sticking in the throat, coughing during meals, and difficulty swallowing.[7,20,23] This checklist of potential problems was used in order to assign patients into symptomatic or asymptomatic groups in our 1991 study and was also used on a long-term basis to evaluate whether patients maintained improved swallowing performance after dysphagia treatment.[23]

INSTRUMENTAL DIAGNOSTIC PROCEDURES

The swallow can be separated into several phases that can be evaluated by means of various radiographic imaging techniques. The videofluoroscopic technique is the most commonly used procedure to evaluate the oropharyngeal swallow: swallowing is examined in relation to the movement of the bolus from the mouth to the stomach. The swallow is usually discussed as having four phases, which occur in rapid succession or overlap in continuous swallowing. In the oral preparatory phase, food is positioned in the mouth and masticated into a swallow-ready bolus resting on the tongue blade. In the oral phase, the bolus is transported posteriorly over the tongue to the area of the anterior faucial arch, where the swallow response is triggered, the palate elevates, and the pharyngeal phase begins. In the pharyngeal phase, the bolus is moved through the pharynx by a combination of gravity and pharyngeal contractions. In the esophageal phase, the upper esophageal sphincter relaxes and opens, allowing the bolus to enter the esophagus, where peristaltic activity transports the material into the stomach.

Although the oral and pharyngeal phases are usually most affected by weak oral and pharyngeal muscles, polio patients can exhibit abnormality in any phase of swallowing. A variety of signs of abnormality an be detected from the videofluoroscopic study. The most common findings have been compiled from several sources[5,7,15,20,23] and are displayed in Table 2, in which specific signs of dysphagia are categorized in regard to the four phases of swallowing: oral preparatory, oral, pharyngeal, and esophageal. In Table 2, the symptoms followed by an asterisk are most likely to cause dysphagia complaints. These symptoms—individually or in combination with one another—may predict aspiration or risk for laryngeal penetration during or after the swallow. In the Sonies and Dalakas study, the most common dysphagic symptoms seen on videofluoroscopy were excessive lingual pumping and tongue gestures, uncontrolled bolus flow and unilateral bolus flow with pooling in the valleculae, and pyriform sinuses.[23]

TABLE 2. Major Findings of Videofluoroscopic Swallowing Studies in Post-Polio Patients Compiled from Several Sources[5,7,15,20,24]

Oral Preparatory Phase
Tongue weakness
Tongue incoordination
Lingual hemiparesis
Lingual residue
Palatal residue
Palatal paresis
Impaired bolus control

Oral Phase
Premature bolus leakage before swallow response*
Nasal regurgitation
Delayed swallow response*
Lingual pumping and tongue gestures

Pharyngeal Phase
Delayed swallow response*
Delayed pharyngeal transit
Unilateral pharyngeal weakness
Bilateral pharyngeal weakness*
Unilateral pooling in valleculae
Unilateral pooling in pyriform sinus
Laryngeal penetration*
Silent aspiration*
Aspiration
Delayed hyolaryngeal elevation*
Incomplete laryngeal closure*
Impaired epiglottal tilt

Esophageal Phase
Hiatal hernia
Gastroesophageal reflux*
Esophageal spasm
Zenker's diverticulae

*Risk for aspiration

Bilateral pooling in the pyriform sinus and laryngeal penetration were noted only in patients who were aware of swallowing difficulty. A variety of esophageal symptoms were found in all patients regardless of whether or not they had complaints of dysphagia.

Ultrasound imaging can be used to examine the oral preparatory and oropharyngeal swallow. There is no need to ingest contrast material, and any kind of food can be ingested. It is also possible to evaluate the unstimulated saliva swallow in persons at risk for aspiration. The total duration of the oropharyngeal swallow can be quantified by ultrasound studies. Significant differences have been found in the duration of swallowing a water bolus between symptomatic and asymptomatic polio patients on ultrasound.[23] This finding suggests that extra effort was required because of lingual and pharyngeal weakness in the symptomatic group.

PROGRESSION OF OROPHARYNGEAL SYMPTOMS

"Postpoliomyelitis state [can be viewed] as a continuum, starting with those who have mild and stable compromise, through those with ongoing musculoskeletal symptoms and extending to those who have new weakness (PPMA), [rather] than as a state comprising distinct subgroups" (p. 18).[18] This does not indicate that all patients will progress at the same rate or have the same symptoms. It does, however, suggest that patients who have symptoms of dysphagia caused by weak oral pharyngeal musculature are at greater risk for developing additional signs of progression of dysphagia. If muscle function in the oropharynx or larynx were to worsen below a presently undetermined threshold, then ability to execute a swallowing response would most likely change. Certainly this must be a valid supposition or there would be few patients complaining of new symptoms of dysphagia.

In order to test the argument, we recalled four patients at random from our original 32 patients and repeated all of the original measures. In all of these patients the original signs of dysphagia had progressed. Two patients who were originally unaware of swallowing difficulty became aware of problems. One patient remained unaware of difficulty in spite of displaying more severe pharyngeal and esophageal signs. Since that time, more patients have returned for follow-up studies and all have some indications of changes in bolus transport or initiation of swallowing. None of our patients have aspirated to date. We believe this is due to their compliance with our therapy suggestions. All patients are counseled at each evaluation regarding individual strategies for swallowing safety and included in short-term treatment as appropriate. Certainly there is agreement that an individual will benefit from dysphagia treatment tailored to that individual's specific patterns.[6] Although physiological signs of dysfunction may exacerbate, continual evaluation and revision of treatment plans for dysphagia can reduce serious risk of aspiration in most patients.

DISCUSSION AND SUMMARY

Post-poliomyelitis has caused a variety of signs of oropharyngeal dysfunction in patients with an original diagnosis of bulbar polio. Speech, voice, respiration, and swallowing may be impaired in these individuals. It is not surprising that PPMA will cause progression of these symptoms and a worsening of the ability to swallow. However, in patients without previous speech or swallowing difficulty whose original diagnosis was nonbulbar poliomyelitis, new signs of dysphagia may emerge several decades after the original episode and may progress. Because of the various compensatory motions that can occur to accommodate changes in the oropharyngeal musculature, many persons remain unaware that they have sustained any deficits in speaking or swallowing until symptoms have become moderate in degree. It is likely that abnormalities in bulbar neurons emerge in the same slowly progressive manner as in the limb muscles.

Long-term monitoring of speech and swallowing behavior using objective methods may help in charting progressing of disease. Periodic dynamic imaging studies using videofluoroscopy and ultrasound should be used to monitor progression of symptoms and to provide the information needed to modify treatment strategies. Dysphagia and speech therapy techniques are an essential component of long-term assessment and treatment for post-polio patients. Whereas other symptoms that have been described, such as leg pain, muscle weakness, and fatigue, are notable, they are not likely to cause serious health care problems or affect longevity. In contrast, the worsening of oropharyngeal function can cause impairments in swallowing function, leading to the more serious problem of aspiration pneumonia, which shortens the life span.

At the present time, no large, long-term studies are examining the incidence of new or worsening dysphagic complaints. We are uncertain whether or not small amounts of aspirated material ingested into the lungs over long periods of time will produce cumulative deficits of a serious nature, and research must be conducted to best meet the needs of survivors of the polio epidemic.

REFERENCES

1. Agre JC, Grimby G, Einarsson G, et al: A comparison between post-polio individuals in Sweden and the United States [abstract]. Arch Phys Med Rehabil 74:1261, 1993.
2. Bosma JF: Studies of disability of the pharynx resultant from poliomyelitis. Ann Otol Rhinol Laryngol 62:529–547, 1953.
3. Bruno RL, Frick NM: The psychology of polio as a prelude to post-polio sequela: Behavior modification and psychotherapy. Orthopedics 14:1169–1170, 1991.
4. Buchholz DW: Dysphagia in post-polio patients. In Halstead DS, Wichers DO, eds: Research and Clinical Aspects of the Late Effects of Poliomyelitis. Birth Defects 23(4):51–61, 1987.
5. Buchholz DW, Jones B: Dysphagia occurring after polio. Arch Phys Med Rehabil 72:13, 1991.
6. Buchholz DW, Jones B: Post-polio dysphagia: Alarm or caution? Orthopedics 14:12, 1991.
7. Coelho CA, Ferranti R: Incidence and nature of dysphagia in polio survivors. Arch Phys Med Rehabil 72:1071–1075, 1991.
8. Dalakas MC; Dysphagia in the post-polio syndrome [letter and comment] N Engl J Med 325:1107–1109, 1991.
9. Dalakas MC: Morphological changes in the muscles of patients with post-poliomyelitis neuromuscular symptoms. Neurology 38:99–104, 1988.
10. Dalakas MC: New neuromuscular symptoms in patients with old poliomyelitis: A three-year follow up study. Eur Neurol 25:381, 1986.
11. Dalakas MC: Post-polio syndrome. Curr Opin Rheumatol 2:901, 1990.
12. Dalakas MC, Elder G, Hallett M, et al: A long-term follow-up study of patients with post-poliomyelitis neuromuscular symptoms. N Engl J Med 314:959, 1986.
13. Dalakas MC, Hallett M: The post-polio syndrome. In Plum F, ed: Advances in Contemporary Neurology. Philadelphia, F.A. Davis 1988, pp 51–94.
14. Halstead LS: Assessment and differential diagnosis for post-polio syndrome. Orthopedics 14:1209–1217, 1991.
15. Jones B, Buchholz DW, Ravich WJ, Donner MW: Swallowing dysfunction in the post polio syndrome: A cinefluorographic study. AJR 158:2, 1992.
16. Peach PE, Olejnik S: Effect of treatment and noncompliance on post-polio sequelae. Orthopedics 14:1199–1203, 1991.
17. Ramlow J, Alexander M, LaPorte R, et al: Epidemiology of post-polio syndrome. Am J Epidemiol 136:769–786, 1992.
18. Ravits J, Hallett M, Baker M, et al: Clinical and electromyographic studies of post-poliomyelitis muscular atrophy. Muscle Nerve 13:667–674, 1990.
19. Scheer J, Luborsky ML: The cultural context of polio biographies. Orthopedics 14:1173–1187, 1991.
20. Silbergleit AK, Waring WP, Sullivan MJ, Maynard FM: Evaluation, treatment, and follow-up results of post polio patients with dysphagia. Otolaryngol Head Neck Surg 104:333–338, 1991.
21. Sonies, BC: The aging oropharyngeal system. In Ripich DN (ed): Handbook of Geriatric Communication Disorders. Austin, TX, Pro-ed, 1991, pp 187–204.
22. Sonies, BC: Oropharyngeal dyspgagia in the elderly. Clin Geriatr Med 8(3):569–577, 1992.

23. Sonies BC, Dalakas MC: Dysphagia in patients with the post-polio syndrome: N Engl J Med 324:1162–1167, 1991.

24. Sonies BC, Dalakas MC: Swallowing and post-polio. Presented at the annual meeting of American Academy of Neurology, Cincinnati, Ohio, 1988.

25. Sonies BC, Parent LJ, Morrish K, Baum BJ: Durational aspects of the oral-pharyngeal phase of swallow in normal adults. Dysphagia 3:1–10, 1988.

26. Sonies BC, Weiffenbach J, Atkinson J, et al: Clinical examination of motor and sensory functions of the adult oral cavity. Dysphagia 1:178–186, 1987.

27. Tomlinson BE, Irving D: Changes in spinal cord motor neurons of possible relevance to the late effects of poliomyelitis. In Halstead LS, Wiechers DO (eds): Late Effects of Poliomyelitis. Miami, Symposia Foundation, 1985, pp 57–70.

28. Windebank AJ, Litchy WJ, Daube JR, et al: Late effects of paralytic poliomyelitis in Olmsted County, Minnesota. Neurology 41:501–507, 1991.

APPENDIX A

Speech-Language Pathology Swallowing Questionnaire

Ratings: 1—normal   none   never
         2—mild   a little   occasionally
         3—moderate   a fair bit   often
         4—severe   lots   usually–always

1. Does saliva collect in your mouth?	1	2	3	4
2. Do you notice drooling during the day?	1	2	3	4
3. Do you notice drooling at night?	1	2	3	4
4. Do you cough, choke, or awaken with nighttime secretions?	1	2	3	4
5. Do you have difficulty swallowing liquids?	1	2	3	4
6. Do you have difficulty swallowing purees or soft or sticky food (mashed potatoes, rice, puddings)?	1	2	3	4
7. Do you have difficulty swallowing solids (meat, raw vegetables)?	1	2	3	4
8. Have you eliminated any foods from your diet because of difficulty swallowing?	1	2	3	4
9. Do you have excessive saliva?	1	2	3	4
10. Do you have dry mouth?	1	2	3	4
11. Are you a fast eater?	1	2	3	4
12. Are you a slow eater?	1	2	3	4
13. Has your taste sensation (for sweet, bitter, salty, sour, etc.) changed?	1	2	3	4
14. Do you experience discomfort with hot or cold temperatures?	1	2	3	4
15. Do you experience discomfort with spicy food?	1	2	3	4
16. Do you have difficulty chewing hard food (hard candy, raw vegetables)?	1	2	3	4
17. Does food spread all over your mouth: does it pocket in your cheeks?	1	2	3	4
18. Does food or liquid ever come up through your nose?	1	2	3	4
19. Does food or do pills ever stick in your throat?	1	2	3	4
20. Do you experience heartburn/indigestion?	1	2	3	4
21. Does food or liquid ever back up into your mouth?	1	2	3	4
22. Do you ever cough when you eat?	1	2	3	4
23. Have you had episodes of choking or airway obstruction when eating?	1	2	3	4
24. Do you experience upper respiratory problems such as pneumonia or bronchitis?	1	2	3	4
25. Do you have pain when swallowing?	1	2	3	4

NAME: _____   AGE: _____
DATE: _____   SEX: _____

Check the statements that describe you:
1. _____ difficulty swallowing
2. _____ pain while swallowing
3. _____ "lump" in throat
4. _____ can't chew hard foods
5. _____ can't chew fibrous or "crunchy" foods
6. _____ avoid foods like applies, nuts, and cookies
7. _____ avoid foods like celery
8. _____ food spreads all over mouth while eating
9. _____ food gets caught in cheek and is not swallowed
10. _____ food falls out of mouth before swallowing
11. _____ excessive saliva or mucus in mouth
12. _____ very dry mouth
13. _____ food comes out of mouth, or nose while swallowing
14. _____ cough or choke before, during, or after swallowing
15. _____ food gets caught at base of tongue, high in throat
16. _____ food gets caught lower in throat
17. _____ slow eater
18. _____ food or water comes into mouth without vomiting, often while lying down
19. _____ more difficulty swallowing liquids than solids
20. _____ more difficulty swallowing solids than liquids
21. _____ difficulty swallowing pills

Do you have:
1. _____ poor fitting dentures
2. _____ dry mouth (xerostomia)
3. _____ frequent heartburn or indigestion
4. _____ hoarseness after swallowing
5. _____ decreased oral sensation
6. _____ paralysis of oral or facial muscles
7. _____ frequent pneumonia or respiratory problems

Have you been told you have:
1. _____ dysphagia
2. _____ hiatal hernia
3. _____ gastric or peptic ulcer
4. _____ thyroid disorder
5. _____ amyotrophic lateral scelerosis (ALS)
6. _____ multiple sclerosis (MS)
7. _____ Parkinson's disease
8. _____ muscular dystrophy
9. _____ dystonia
10. _____ myasthenia gravis
11. _____ dermatomyositis

12. _____ scleroderma
13. _____ rheumatoid arthritis
14. _____ cerebral palsy
15. _____ poliomyelitis
16. _____ dysautonomia
17. _____ Raynaud's phenomenon (hands or feet turn red or blue)
18. _____ schizophrenia or other psychiatric disorder
19. _____ stroke
20. _____ cancer of the lips, mouth, throat, larynx, or neck
21. _____ structural abnormality of the face or mouth
22. _____ cleft lip/palate
23. _____ polymyositis
24. _____ diabetes

Have you ever had:
1. _____ surgery or radiation to the thyroid
2. _____ surgery or radiation of the face, head, neck or mouth
3. _____ head trauma
4. _____ brain surgery
5. _____ cardiac surgery
6. _____ high blood pressure

Have you taken or do you take:
1. _____ tranquilizers
2. _____ antacids
3. _____ cancer drugs
4. _____ ulcer drugs
5. _____ heart medications
6. _____ insulin

List all other medication you currently take (other than vitamins):

Food preferences/history:

Foods you avoid:

Foods you prefer:

9

Strategies for Exercise Prescription in Post-Polio Patients

ANNE CARRINGTON GAWNE, MD

Appropriate exercises have been shown to improve muscular strength and endurance, improve range of motion, and reduce functional deficits associated with many disabilities. In dealings with the patient with a history of polio, however, several questions arise: How much exercise is enough, and when is it too much? What kinds of exercise are best? What kinds of exercise may be harmful? And are there any guidelines to prescribe a safe and effective exercise program? To answer these questions, it is helpful to first understand the basic principles of exercise physiology, as well as the pathophysiology involved in post-polio syndrome. Following a discussion of these issues is a review of the literature on the effects of exercise in neurologically intact and post-polio individuals. Finally, a new classification system is presented, which will facilitate the prescription of exercise regimens that are both safe and effective in this population.

MUSCLE EXERCISE PHYSIOLOGY

The effects of exercise are seen at two levels. The first is the cellular level, or in the muscle fiber. The second is throughout the cardiovascular and **141** respiratory systems to meet the physiologic demands of the muscle fibers. The two are discussed separately, looking first at muscle strength and then at cardiovascular endurance.

Muscular strength is the maximal force that can be exerted by a muscle.[21] An **isometric contraction** is one in which tension develops but in which the muscle stays the same length.[48] An **isotonic contraction,** or, more appropriately, a dynamic contraction, is one in which the muscle shortens (concentric) or lengthens (eccentric) against a constant resistance, with the muscle tension varying somewhat throughout the range of motion.[24,48] An **isokinetic contraction** is one in which the tension, developed by the muscle as it shortens, is maximal at all joint angles over the full range of motion and in which the velocity remains constant.[56]

When the three types of contractions are compared, the isokinetic one theoretically leads to the greatest improvements in both strength and endurance because it activates a larger number of motor units.[56] However, because it requires special equipment and trained personnel to administer, it is much less readily available. Significant strength gains occur with both eccentric and concentric contractions, and exercise equipment to perform these contractions is easy to find and affordable.[23] The advantages of isometric exercises are limited as the development of strength and endurance is specific to the joint angle at which the muscle is trained. Isometric exercises do have a place with individuals who have joints immobilized secondary to surgery or casting.

The overload principle states that muscles increase in size and strength when forced to contract at tensions close to their maximum.[46] Physiologic changes accompanying increased strength include hypertrophy—the increase in cross-sectional area of the muscle fibers. Hypertrophy is attributable to one or more of the following changes: increased number of myofibrils per muscle fiber; increased protein, especially in the myosin filament; increased capillary density per fiber; increased amounts and strength of connective tissue; and increased number of fibers from longitudinal fiber splitting.[48] These morphologic changes are seen more frequently with eccentric contractions.

Additional factors responsible for strength gains are central nervous system (CNS) adaptations. These include an increase in the number of motor units activated, an increase in the rate of activation, and increased synchronization of motor unit firing.[56] Such changes occur at the spinal cord level and are responsible for cross-education, a phenomenon seen commonly in a limb contralateral to the trained limb. In general, younger individuals (18–26 years old) increase their muscle strength due to hypertrophy, whereas strength gains by older individuals (67–72 years old) are predominantly due to CNS adaptations.[49,50]

Atrophy, or the reduction in size of a muscle, occurs with denervation or when an extremity is placed at rest. Morphological changes seen after a muscle has been immobilized include atrophy of type I muscle fibers, whereas atrophy associated with aging is predominantly limited to a decrease in type II fiber area.[56]

PATHOPHYSIOLOGY IN POST-POLIO MUSCLES

In patients with a history of polio, additional changes occur and there is frequently the development of new weakness and atrophy in muscles both affected and apparently unaffected by the virus.[14,18,19,38–40,47] This phenomenon was clinically observed as early as 1917, when Lovett described progressive upper extremity weakness in men with a history of polio who performed farmwork on a daily basis.[47] In the 1950s, Bennett and Knowlton described a similar overuse weakness.[10] More recently, this new weakness has been termed "post-polio muscular atrophy" (PPMA) or "post-polio syndrome" (PPS).[19,40] The etiology of these changes remains uncertain; however, many feel that it is due to overuse.[6,13,15,16,44,53,55,61] At the time of the initial infection there is loss of anterior horn cell nerve terminals with reinnervation by the sprouting of the remaining motor neurons. As a result there is an increase in motor unit territory, and greater requirements are placed on the remaining fibers, stressing the metabolic demands. If the remaining fibers are unable to meet these demands, a slow deterioration may develop, with resulting new weakness and atrophy. In addition to an overuse phenomenon, new weakness may develop due to disuse.[6,35]

Common morphological changes have also been described in muscles with a history of polio. Dalakas et al. evaluated a population of 27 post-polio patients and documented new weakness over an 8-year period.[19] Biopsy findings at follow-up included changes in cell morphology, fiber type grouping, small angulated fibers, and hypertrophy of muscles that were less affected. Grimby et al. demonstrated that morphologic changes seen in patients with post-polio weakness include an increase in fiber area with hypertrophy and an increase in percentage of type I fibers in the weakest or more overused muscles.[27,34,35] Borg et al. also documented an increased percentage in type I fibers. In addition, internal nuclei and fiber splitting were prominent findings.[13]

As a result, a controversy arises about the role of exercise in the individual with a history of polio. Though many of the morphologic findings are actually similar to changes seen in normal muscle, the lack of sufficient reserve places the polio-weakened muscle at risk for further weakness should overuse occur. Following is a review of the literature on exercise in neurologically intact and polio-affected individuals to gain a better understanding of these concepts.

EFFECTS OF STRENGTH-TRAINING PROGRAMS IN NEUROLOGICALLY INTACT INDIVIDUALS

One of the first formal isotonic strengthening programs was described in 1948 by Delorme and Watkins.[23] They introduced the term "progressive resistance exercise" (PRE) and the concept of the ten repetition maximum (10 RM)—the maximum load a muscle group can lift ten times. For each muscle group to be trained, the exercise program consisted of a total of 30 repetitions, divided into three sets of ten as follows:

set 1 = 10 repetitions at 50% 10 RM
set 2 = 10 repetitions at 75% 10 RM
set 3 = 10 repetitions at 100% 10 RM

Delorme and Watkins recommended the training frequency to be 4 consecutive days per week and were able to show demonstrable gains using this program. Isometric programs have also demonstrated that strength can be gained or maintained with a few maximal contractions held for 5–10 seconds three to five times per week.[41]

EFFECTS OF STRENGTH-TRAINING PROGRAMS IN POST-POLIO INDIVIDUALS

Many studies that have looked at the effect of strengthening exercises from a few weeks to a few years after the acute episode of polio demonstrated that these exercises are responsible for many of the gains in strength seen after the initial episode. In 1948, Delorme and colleagues applied the principle of PREs to 19 post-polio patients.[22] The patients had a history of polio from 1 to 49 years previously. They exercised once daily, 4 days a week, with 10 RM recalculated weekly. Twenty-seven muscle groups were evaluated, and of these, 17 demonstrated gross gains in strength (an increase in the muscle grade) measured with manual muscle testing (MMT). Muscle power in 15 of 27 quadriceps muscles doubled or more than doubled as measured by a spring scale. All except three muscles showed an increase in work capacity. It was noted that the largest improvements were seen in those muscle groups that had begun with greater than antigravity (fair plus) strength. Functional improvements included the ability to perform ordinary activities with less effort and fatigue. Delorme et al. stressed the importance of not putting too much emphasis on MMT alone; therefore, they used the spring scale to quantify strength more accurately. Evidence for functional improvement, however, was largely anecdotal.

Gurewitsch evaluated 13 patients who were in the initial phases of recovery from their polio in 1950.[36] They exercised all but the very weak muscles, with a modification of the protocol of Delorme et al., six to eight times daily, until they reached a state of fatigue. Strength was monitored by MMT. When they reached the point where they could do 20–30 repetitions easily, the exercise load was increased. Both muscle strength and endurance increased 50%. However, care was taken not to increase the workload too rapidly. Gureswitsch recognized that severely affected, atrophic muscles were not appropriate for strengthening. He did not quantify strength or fatigue objectively, which leads to concern, given such a strenuous protocol.

When PPMA was first widely recognized in the early 1980s, additional exercise studies were designed. The investigations included survivors many years after their initial episode of polio and in general demonstrated similar results.

In 1984, Feldman and Soskolne developed an exercise protocol they described as "nonfatiguing strengthening exercises" for a population of six patients with post-polio symptoms.[28,29] They initially evaluated 32 sets of muscles by electromyography (EMG) and assessed strength with a myometer. They described EMG features of absence of insertional activity, normal-appearing motor unit action potentials (MUAPs) with polyphasic potentials, and a decreased interference pattern. The protocol began using 50% of the maximum weight that could be lifted five times (5 RM). The patient began with five repetitions, then gradually increased to 30 repetitions. At this point, the weight was increased to 75% of the original 5 RM. Again the patient started with five repetitions, increasing to 30. The gradual progression was increased until the patient started with five repetitions, increasing to 30. The gradual progression was increased until the patient reached the point where further progression caused fatigue. This was performed three times weekly for a period of 3–6 months. The investigators found that by using this routine for at least 24 weeks, 14 muscles (46%) got stronger, as measured by myometry, 17 (53%) showed no change, and one muscle got weaker. There was no relationship between the degree of initial weakness and improvement in strength. Problems with this study include lack of a clear definition of post-polio syndrome and the description of the EMG changes (normal MUAPs is not a common finding). In addition, the authors did not define the mode in which the repetitions were performed (e.g., continuous versus sets), and there were no controls.

Einarsson and Grimby developed an exercise program in 1987 for 12 post-polio patients, nine of whom had symptoms of PPS.[26] These patients were all walkers with at least 3/5 strength in their quadriceps muscle. Muscle strength was evaluated on a Cybex dynamometer, and muscle biopsies were done before and after training. The training protocol used a warm-up period followed by three sets of eight alternating isokinetic and isometric exercises for a total of 6 weeks. The program was completed without discomfort or evidence of ill effects. Only one leg was trained; the other served as a control. There was a significant strength gain in the trained leg that persisted even past the end of the training period. Follow-up biopsy showed increased fiber area in five of seven patients; however, changes in muscle strength did not correlate significantly with changes in muscle fiber size. This study was notable for performing biopsies to confirm histologically the presence of old polio and for using objective quantitative measurements. The authors did not specify, however, which of the muscles (those with or without new weakness) showed improvement. Use of the contralateral leg as a control is problematic, since many times they are not equally affected. The investigators concluded that increases in strength might be explained through both muscular and neural adaptations.

In 1991, Einarsson described a similar protocol used for muscle conditioning in 30 post-polio patients.[25] These patients had at least 3/5 strength in their quadriceps and a history of polio at least 25 years previously. Muscle strength measurements of knee flexion and extension both isometrically and isokinetically were done initially and at 6 and 12 months. Muscle biopsies confirmed the presence of polio. The program consisted of a warm-up period followed by 12 sets of eight isokinetic knee extension contractions at 180°/s alternating with 12 sets of 4-second isometric contractions. This was performed three times a week for 6 weeks. The knee flexors were not exercised and therefore acted as a control. There was a significant improvement (24%) in knee extension strength, with no change in the strength of the knee flexors. These changes were also associated with subjective positive changes in functional tasks and general well-being. Although functional changes were noted, they were not quantified, and the location of new weakness was not specified.

In that same year, Fillyaw used Delorme's training program on 17 patients who had EMG evidence of polio, muscle strength of fair or above, and evidence of PPS.[30] The quadriceps or biceps was exercised, with the contralateral extremity used as a control. Three sets of ten repetitions with a 5-minute rest between sets were performed every other day. The 10 RM was recalculated every 2 weeks. The patients were instructed to stop if they experienced pain or fatigue. Maximum isotonic torque was measured initially, then every 3 months for 2 years. Sixteen of 17 patients demonstrated significant strength gains, but there was no evidence of increased endurance. The researchers cautioned that the patients undergo periodic quantitative muscle testing under the supervision of a physical therapist to avoid overwork weakness. This study and its method are notable, for they use quantitative measures of both strength and endurance as guidelines, and they test muscles with EMG to verify the presence of old polio.

More recently, Agre and colleagues used a 12-week isotonic strengthening program in subjects with at least fair plus quadriceps strength.[6] The subjects exercised with sandbag weights attached to their ankles, performing six to ten knee extensions holding the weight for 5 seconds, then resting for 25 seconds. This was increased until the patient could perform ten repetitions with a perceived exertion of "very hard" according to Borg's rating of perceived exertion (RPE). In 12 weeks, the average weight that each subject could lift more than doubled. There were neither EMG changes nor an increase in creatine phosphokinase over this time. This study used readily available equipment and quantitative measures of exertion, and it documents that a carefully supervised exercise program can safely increase strength in this population.[1]

Agre and Rodriquez have also described an exercise technique known as "pacing", mixing periods of exercise with periods of rest, in post-polio patients[2-5] (*see also* Chapter 4). The presence of polio was confirmed by EMG testing, and all measurements were done with objective quantitative measurements. In summary, Agre and Rodriquez evaluated symptomatic polio subjects (those complaining of progressive loss of strength) and tested them on three separate days, at least a week apart.[5] Parameters collected included maximum strength, endurance, work capacity, and time for recovery on an exhausting exercise done with the quadriceps. The authors also measured isometric quadriceps strength during a 3-second maximal volitional contraction (MVC). On the first day, the subject performed a quadriceps contraction at 40% MVC until exhaustion, waited 30 seconds, and then performed a 5-second MVC trial. On the second day, the subject exercised in quartiles with a 2-minute rest between trials. Finally, on the third day, the subject contracted the quadriceps muscle at 40% of MVC for 20 seconds and had a 2-minute rest break, for a total of 18 sessions. The investigators discovered that when the subject paced himself (day 3), there was less evidence of muscle fatigue, increased capacity to perform work, and increased ability to recover strength after activity. The total amount of work done was greatest (237%) on day 3. This study utilized the concept of the RPE as a way to avoid overfatigue. The principle of pacing has been applied only to isometric contraction of one muscle group in individuals known to have at least 3/5 strength and has not been well studied in an exercise program involving the whole body. Nonetheless, the authors successfully specified and compared the results of training programs for muscles that are both getting weaker and remaining stable.

Regarding the long-term safety of an exercise program, most studies are limited at the present time, because they were initiated only within the past few years. Because less objective measures of muscle strength were used in the past, previous studies are less valuable, and manual muscle testing has been shown to be unreliable in comparison to more quantitative measurements, especially in the good to normal range.[3,9,22,43] Dalakas demonstrated a loss of strength in polio patients over a 3-year period using MMT.[18] But Agre and Rodriguez evaluated a group of patients after 1 year and 3 years, using objective quantifiable measurements of muscle strength (peak isometric and isokinetic force) and found no significant strength losses on follow-up[5] (*see also* chapter 4). Munsat followed 44 patients from 400 to 2,100 days using a quantitative isometric measurement—the Tufts quantitative neuromuscular exam—and demonstrated no significant deterioration in muscle force.[52]

More evidence supporting findings of long-term strength gains in affected muscle was demonstrated in a study done by Munin et al.[51] They studied seven patients with quadriceps strength less than 5/5, recent weakness and generalized fatigue on one side, and a contralateral muscle of normal strength without new weakness. They tested patients' strength using an isokinetic/isometric protocol. They consistently saw no decline in strength on either side over a 3-year period. In fact, the strength actually increased. However, all their patients had at least 3/5 strength in the affected quadriceps, and none were older than 60. Unfortunately, neither EMG nor biopsies were performed either to confirm or rule out the presence of anterior horn cell disease in either extremity.

It is the consensus of most authors that quantifiable measures of strength, endurance, and degree of involvement with polio are needed to follow more accurately the long-term effects of an exercise program. A laboratory test (either an EMG or biopsy) also should be performed to either confirm or rule out the presence of polio. In addition, it is imperative to state whether the muscles that are being exercised have symptoms of new weakness.

EFFECTS OF CARDIOVASCULAR TRAINING PROGRAMS IN NEUROLOGICALLY INTACT INDIVIDUALS

Muscular endurance is defined as the ability of a muscle group to perform repeated contractions against a light load for an extended period of time. Cardiovascular endurance describes the ability to perform a sustained activity for an extended period of time and depends on efficient respiratory and cardiovascular systems. Normal changes seen with exercise include an increase in the maximal O_2 consumption (VO_2 max) accomplished through a combination of factors. There is an increase in stroke volume (SV) with greater cardiac contractibility and efficiency as well as an increase in blood volume and percentage of hemoglobin. Within the lungs there is an increase in vital capacity (VC) and inspiratory capacity. Subsequently, with training, the heart rate per work load decreases so the individual can perform work with less stress. Secondary effects of exercise include increased coronary blood flow due to increased collateral circulation and a decrease in the resting heart rate and blood pressure.[24,56]

A commonly used measure of energy use is the MET, or metabolic equivalent. One MET is equal to the basal energy requirement while sitting and awake (3.5 mL/kg · min). As energy expenditure increases, the MET increases in a linear fashion.[56] Table 1 lists the approximate METs in both activities of daily living (ADLs) and exercise activities.

Another important tool used in exercise prescription is the RPE developed by Borg.[11,12] This is a scale on which perceived exertion is quantified on a numerical scale, with 6 being very very light and 20 being very, very hard. The American College of Sports Medicine (ACSM) has modified this scale using a 1–10 system (Table 2).[8]

The ACSM has also established minimal guidelines including frequency, intensity, and duration of exercise needed in order to obtain a training effect. Recommended frequency is three or four times per week, duration is 20–30 minutes, and intensity is 70–80% of the person's VO_2 max.[9] In addition, the ACSM recommends the following components for any exercise program: warm-up, stretching, exercise, cool down.

EFFECTS OF CARDIOVASCULAR TRAINING PROGRAMS IN POST-POLIO INDIVIDUALS

In 1987, Alba et al. evaluated the work capacity of 35 patients—20 females and 15 males—33 of whom were complaining of new symptoms, in order

TABLE 1. Table of Metabolic Equivalents (METS)

1.5–2 METS	Doing seated ADLs (eating, facial hygiene, resting) Doing seated recreation (sewing, playing cards, painting) Doing seated occupational activities (writing, typing, clerical work)
2–3 METS	Standing ADLs (dressing, showering, shaving, light housework) Standing occupation (mechanic, bartender, auto repair) Standing recreation (fishing, billiards, shuffleboard) Walking 2.5 mph Bike riding 5–6 mph
4–5 METS	Doing heavy housework (scrubbing floor, hanging wash) Canoeing, golfing, playing softball, playing tennis, badminton (doubles) Social dancing, cross-country hiking Swimming 20 yd/min Walking 4 mph (level), (3 mph on 5% grade) Bike riding 10 mph
6–7 METS	Heavy gardening (digging dirt, lawn mowing, hoeing) Skating, water-skiing Playing tennis, badminton (singles) Stair-climbing (<27 ft/min) Swimming 25 yd/min Walking 5 mph (level) (3.5 MPH on 5% grade)
8–9 METS	Active occupation (sawing wood, digging ditches, shoveling snow) Active recreation (downhill skiing, ice hockey, paddleball) Bike riding 12–14 mph Stair-climbing (27 ft/min) Swimming 35 yd/min Walking 9 mph (level) (3 mph on 15% grade) Jogging 5–6 mph

Data compiled from numerous sources.[8,56]

to determine their cardiovascular status.[7] The patients performed a graded exercise test using an arm ergometer, a chair ergometer, and a treadmill according to their ambulatory ability. Parameters evaluated included muscle strength using MMT, body weight, maximum METS, maximum heart rate (HRmax), VO_2 max, and VC. Alba et al. divided the patients into three subgroups: ambulatory without restriction to moderate restriction, ambulatory with moderately severe to severe restriction, and wheelchair bound. Significant findings included greater weakness in the lower extremities than the upper extremities and a decreased VC, especially in those who smoked or had a history of respiratory involvement. There were also a decreased HRmax, decreased maximal cardiac output, and decreased work

TABLE 2. American College of Sports Medicine Rating of Perceived Exertion

Grade	Perceived Exertion
0	Nothing
0.5	Very, very weak
1	Very weak
2	Weak
3	Moderate
4	Somewhat strong
5	Strong
6	
7	Very strong
8	
9	
10	Very, very strong
	Maximal

From American College of Sports Medicine: Guidelines for Exercise Testing and Prescription. Philadelphia, Lea & Febiger, 1986, with permission. (Modified from Borg.[11,12])

capacity (similar to a group of hospitalized patients). Of the three groups, the nonambulatory population was affected most significantly. The researchers recommended that patients partake in any repetitive activity that appealed to them—if it was considered "safe"—and recommended stopping the activity if it caused "undue pain, muscle fatigue or a sense of weakness" that required more than the usual time to recover. Though that study is good because it introduces the idea of different ways to assess cardiovascular fitness depending on ambulatory status, the investigators did not specify the degree of involvement of the exercising muscles being exercised. Neither did they compare differences in modalities in a single individual, thus raising the question of the reliability of comparisons of different kinds of exercise.

In 1985, Owens and Jones evaluated the cardiovascular endurance of 21 patients in an electrocardiogram-monitored, symptom-limited, graded exercise test, using either a bicycle or a hand ergometer.[54] They found that the patients had an average maximum fitness level of 5.6 METS, indicative of severe deconditioning. They proposed an exercise program as follows: intensity of 65–80% of reserve heart rate, a duration of 15–30 minutes, and a frequency of three to five times per week on alternate days. The modality used depended on preserved function. Flexibility and warm-up exercises were recommended before each session. However, the authors did not report the results of this proposed exercise regimen in their documentation.

Dean and Ross examined the effects of a modified exercise program in three post-polio patients in 1988.[20] Each subject met the diagnostic criteria for PPS and was ambulatory without assistive devices. One patient was used as an untrained control while the other two walked on a treadmill three times a week at a submaximal rate for a total of 8 weeks, advancing their walking duration from 22 to 31 minutes. RPE was monitored using a 1–10 scale, and pain was monitored using a 1–4 scale. An attempt was made to keep RPE below 2 and pain below 1 (light). After training, on submaximal testing, both of the trained subjects demonstrated reductions in VO_2, heart rate, blood pressure, RPE, and energy cost at similar work loads when compared to the pretest; the untrained subject showed no change. There was no apparent effect of training on pulmonary function. The mechanism for the change was felt to be both cardiovascular conditioning and muscle adaptation. Although the number of subjects is small, this study has the virtue of clearly quantifying symptoms of pain and perceived exertion.

The following year, Jones and colleagues evaluated cardiorespiratory responses to aerobic training in 16 post-polio patients who participated in a 16-week exercise program.[42] These patients met the following criteria: They had a documented history of polio with subsequent improvement, then a period of stability with new complaints of weakness. They had adequate strength to participate in bicycle ergometry (at least 3/5 in their quadriceps and iliopsoas and 2/5 in their hamstrings and gluteals). Baseline tests, including resting heart rate and blood pressure, HRmax, BPmax, VO_2, and VCO_2 and expiratory volume (Ve), were performed on a bicycle ergometer. Patients were divided into an exercise group and a control group. The first group exercised three times a week, once under the supervision of the therapist, for a period of 15–30 minutes using a predetermined target heart rate as a guide. Within this population were two subgroups, determined by their maximum METS. Those with a maximum less than 6 METS exercised for 2–3 minutes, with a 1-minute rest; those with a maximum greater than 6 METS exercised for 4–5 minutes, with a 1-minute rest. Significant results on posttest included an improvement in the total exercise time, total work per time, VO_2, and Vemax within the exercise group. Though a few subjects dropped out for reasons unrelated to the study, none developed any overuse syndromes or other injury due to their exercise. Problems with this study include that the extent of the initial polio was not documented, and it was not specified whether or not the subjects were using polio-affected muscles to perform their exercise.

In a similar study in 1989, Kriz and colleagues examined the effects of an upper extremity arm ergometry program on 29 subjects with a history of polio who met the following criteria: history of polio with subsequent improvement and stabilization, aged 39–60 years old, and adequate arm strength and torso balance to operate an arm ergometer.[45] The subjects had no cardiovascular medical problems or other, neurological problems and were not already participating in a fitness program. They were divided into an exercise group and a control group. The exercise group participated three times a week in a 16-week training program with 1 day of rest between exercise sessions. The group performed the exercises on an arm ergometer with a heart rate of 70–75% heart rate reserve. The investigators evaluated the following variables: resting heart rate, HRmax, and resting and immediate postexercise blood pressure, as well as exercise time, power, respiratory exchange ratio, respiratory rate, maximum VO_2, VCO_2, and Ve. After the 16-week program, the group that exercised showed significant improvement in VO_2 max, VCO_2max, Vemax, power, and exercise time. None of the patients in the exercise group developed problems with pain or overuse. Again, the report did not document the degree of polio involvement in the exercising extremities. In addition, the authors selected subjects younger than 60 years old and without severe weakness.

SUMMARY

Although it has been reported that individuals with a history of polio may develop new weakness many years after the original episode, it has also been shown that these people can gain both muscle strength and cardiovascular endurance from a well-planned training program. For the strengthening of individual muscle groups, the following criteria appear to be necessary: a history of polio with improvement and stabilization and sufficient strength (3/5) to contract that muscle against gravity. There appear to be positive benefits regardless of whether that muscle group is with or without new weakness. The choice of type of exercise program needs to be developed according to both the needs of the individual and the resources available: An isometric program is of benefit for those who have either a joint immobilized in a cast due to surgery or a fracture, whereas an isotonic program is more appropriate for a home exercise program. An isokinetic program appears to be of great benefit whenever the equipment is available, or when a special need arises, such as for strengthening before or after surgery.

The long-term safety of a strenuous strengthening program on muscle that has been severely affected is not known, but the positive effects of exercise on other systems, including cardiovascular and respiratory systems, are clear. It therefore can be concluded that a carefully monitored program is beneficial in selected individuals with a history of polio. It is also possible that many of the secondary symptoms such as generalized fatigue can be reduced as patients become more conditioned and are able to perform similar amounts of work with less expenditure of energy. An ideal cardiovascular program should both exercise the muscles least affected by polio, in order to get maximum cardiovascular benefits, and avoid overuse or secondary degenerative effects on the more affected extremities. For instance, if the legs are the more involved limbs, then the arms can be used in a more strenuous program; or the legs can be exercised if not seriously involved. The exercise program should be initially supervised by a therapist in order to teach proper techniques, including the monitoring of heart rate and RPE. All individuals who are older or with risk factors for cardiovascular disease such as hypertension, smoking, hypercholesterolemia, or a history of coronary artery disease should first undergo a graded exercise test with cardiac monitoring in order to establish the safety of participating in an exercise program. The type of activity should be one that the participant can enjoy so as to reduce lack of interest and subsequent dropout.

A NEW POST-POLIO MUSCLE CLASSIFICATION FOR EXERCISE PRESCRIPTION

In order to prescribe the safest and most appropriate exercise program for the post-polio patients in our clinic, we have developed a limb-specific muscle classification system, the National Rehabilitation Hospital (NRH) Post-Polio Classification.[32] The purpose of the classification is to create a more standardized set of criteria to document the severity of involvement of the polio. This facilitates communication between the therapists and the physician regarding the specificity of the exercise program, sets standards by which to compare the results of clinical trials, and aids in giving recommendations regarding activity, prognosis, and need for assistive equipment. To classify the muscle, a combination of history, physical exam, and EMG is used. When patients are first evaluated, a complete history and physical are performed by the physician, and the patient is referred for a four-extremity EMG.[37] In addition to an evaluation for specific clinical conditions, a screening examination is performed. It includes nerve conduction studies of bilateral median and sensory nerves and at least three muscles in each extremity.[33] Additional benefits of the EMG to the clinician include the ability to rule out other neurological lesions that may require treatment or need to be considered with prescribing an exercise program.[31,33,37]

Following the EMG, each muscle is classified separately and the limb is classified according to the most severely involved muscle. If contralateral extremities exhibited differences and an exercise program uses both, then the exercise program is prescribed on the basis of the most severely affected extremity. Table 3 summarizes this classification system. Table 4 demonstrates the demographic data on 60 consecutive post-polio patients evaluated in our clinic utilizing these methods. Table 5 shows results of the classification of 240 limbs in those 60 patients using the criteria to fol-

TABLE 3. The National Rehabilitation Hospital (NRH) Post-Polio Muscle Classification

Class I	No clinical polio
Class II	Subclinical polio
Class III	Clinically stable polio
Class IV	Clinically unstable polio
Class V	Severely atrophic polio

Data from Gawne and Halstead.[32]

TABLE 4. Demographic Data on 60 Consecutive Post-Polio Outpatients[33]

Sex (M/F)	22/38
Mean age (range), yrs	53 (22–82)
Mean years post-polio	44 (14–80)

Data from Gawne and Halstead.[32]

TABLE 5. NRH Limb Classification of 60 Consecutive Post-Polio Outpatients

NRH Class	Upper Extremity	Lower Extremity	Total
I	63	6	69
II	20	22	42
III	24	40	64
IV	10	27	37
V	3	25	28
TOTAL	120	120	240

Total of 240 limbs measured. Data from Gawne and Halstead.[32]

FIGURE 1. Distribution of upper extremity limbs by NRH class in 60 consecutive post-polio outpatients.[32]

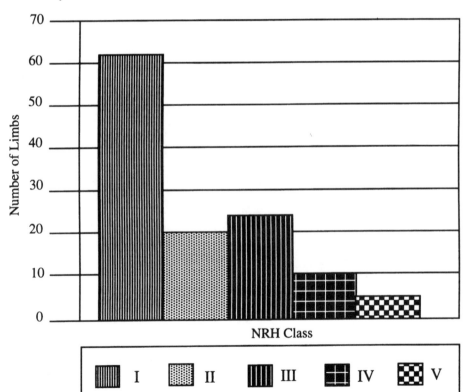

low. The distributions of the findings in both the upper and lower extremities are detailed in Figures 1 and 2. Figure 3 is an algorithm that can be used to aid in this classification process.

NRH Class I muscles (no clinical polio) have no history of past or new weakness. Strength ranges from good to normal, and there is no atrophy or sensory or reflex changes. On EMG there is normal insertional activity, with no evidence of muscle membrane instability such as fibrillation potentials or positive sharp waves. Motor unit action potentials (MUAPs) are normal in size and configuration, with normal recruitment.

The objective of the exercise program for Class I muscles or limbs is to increase muscle strength and cardiovascular endurance. Exercise recommendations consist of an initial set of muscle-stretching exercises to in-

FIGURE 2. Distribution of lower extremity limbs by NRH class in 60 consecutive post-polio outpatients.[32]

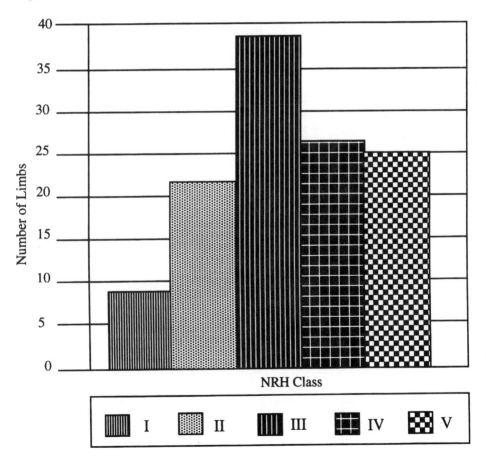

NATIONAL REHABILITATION HOSPITAL POST-POLIO CLASSIFICATION

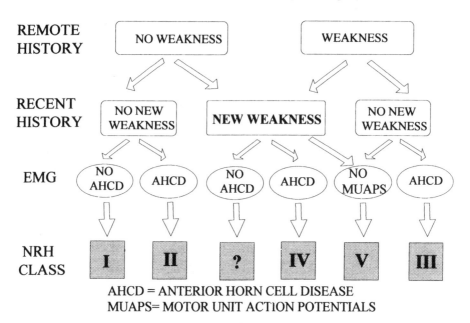

AHCD = ANTERIOR HORN CELL DISEASE
MUAPS= MOTOR UNIT ACTION POTENTIALS

FIGURE 3. NRH post-polio muscle classification. (AHCD—anterior horn cell disease; MUAP—motor unit action potentials.)

crease flexibility, a light warm-up period using the muscles that will be exercised, an exercise program, and, finally, a cool-down period. A strengthening program includes PREs as described by DeLorme,[23] with 1- to 2-minute rest breaks between sets initially. These muscles should be used selectively in order that an aerobic program be able to improve cardiovascular conditioning. When there is no cardiac or respiratory illness, a conditioning program can follow ACSM recommendations for frequency and duration.[8] The ideal frequency of exercise for these extremities should be three or four times a week, for a period of 15–30 minutes at a heart rate of 60–80% of HRmax.[8] Table 1 describes some typical occupational and recreational activities in the 6–9 MET range, which would be appropriate for Class I limbs.

NRH Class II muscles (subclinical polio) have no history of past or new weakness, or, if affected, there was full recovery. Strength is good to normal. Sensation and reflexes are normal. EMG is consistent with anterior horn cell disease. Insertional activity is normal, and there are rarely fibrillations or positive sharp waves. MUAPs are large, with increased polyphasics and decreased recruitment. These muscles probably represent those "unaffected" muscles, previously described by other authors, that eventually get weaker.[14,17,19,57,59,60]

The objectives of the exercise program for Class II extremities are to increase strength in those muscles in the good range and to maintain normal strength in the remainder. If other extremities are more severely affected, Class II extremities can be used to improve cardiovascular endurance. The frequency should be 3 or 4 days a week, for 10–20 minutes. The session should be paced, increasing the frequency of rest breaks until the individual can perform the exercise without significant fatigue either during or after the activity. The frequency of exercise should also be paced, alternating exercise and rest days. As a training effect develops and the individual is able to perform a similar workload with less fatigue, both the amount of resistance used and the frequency and duration of the exercise can be altered to meet the changing increases in strength. But given the threat of PPMA, muscle strength should be monitored to detect overuse weakness early and then decrease the amount of exercise. Maximum activities should be in the 4–7 MET range.

NRH Class III muscles (clinically stable polio) have a remote history of weakness, with some improvement and no complaints of new weakness. On physical examination, the strength ranges from fair to good. Sensation is normal, and reflexes are normal or decreased proportional to the muscle strength and bulk. Atrophy may be present, EMG is consistent with anterior horn cell disease, with normal insertional activity. Sometimes there are fibrillation potentials or positive sharp waves, but generally these are small and sparse. MUAPs are usually larger than those of Class II muscles, with increased polyphasics and decreased recruitment. These muscles represent those previously described as asymptomatic[3]; however, they are now frequently referred to as clinically stable, as suggested by Grimby.

The goals for class III extremities are to at least maintain strength and, if possible, to gain strength in those muscles that are deconditioned. Exercise recommendations include active range of motion (AROM) or passive range of motion (PROM), depending on the strength of the muscle. Strengthening exercises are similar to those in Class II, with further modifications made for pacing and for the exercising of muscles with less than antigravity strength. A typical set of PREs as Feldman has described or an isokinetic program as Einarrson described would also be appropriate. Strength should be carefully monitored and the program modified if weakness develops. Because of weakness and susceptibility to stresses with weight bearing in extremities with degenerative joint disease, non-weight-bearing exercises such as a pool program are preferred. An aerobic program should be paced at a submaximal heart rate. Activities in the 2–5 MET range would be appropriate.

NRH Class IV muscles (clinically unstable polio) are either those that are developing new weakness and atrophy (PPMA) or those previously described as symptomatic.[3] They are weaker, with less dynamic and isometric strength than those in Class III. Sensation is normal, atrophy usually is present, and reflexes are decreased. EMG findings are similar to Class III; however, MUAP amplitude and polyphasics may be increased.[3] Recruitment may be less,[57] and there may be more significant new denervation fibrillations, positive sharp waves.[32,53]

The main goal in this class is to prevent further weakness, so it is recommended first to decrease activity if overuse is suspected. If disuse is suspected or rest does not help, then an exercise program is begun. Exercise recommendations include PROM or AROM. A nonfatiguing exercise program would be appropriate for strengthening. Because many muscles may have less than antigravity strength, exercises should be done in a gravity-eliminated position or in a pool. Muscle strength is carefully monitored. This program should be done no more than three times a week and should be modified if symptoms of pain, new weakness, or fatigue develop. For cardiovascular conditioning, we generally recommend it be used in ADLs only (1–3 METS). As we have found that many of our patients have less affected upper extremities (Figs. 1 and 2), we frequently advise such patients to do a cardiovascular exercise using only their arms, such as swimming or arm ergometry. For those limbs with severe weakness, we recommend avoiding weight bearing by use of assistive devices or a wheelchair or motorized scooter. Bracing is needed for those lower extremities with less than antigravity strength.

NRH Class V muscles (severely atrophic polio) are those that are originally affected, with severe weakness and little improvement. New weakness may be present; however, the muscle is already so weak it is hard to tell if there is new weakness. On physical examination, they are extremely weak (trace to poor), with marked atrophy, no sensory changes, and areflexia. On EMG there are decreased insertional activity; few fibrillation or positive sharp waves; little to no MUAPs, with variable amplitude; increased polyphasics; and markedly decreased recruitment. This class is similar to Dalakas's group 1, with morphological features of fibrosis, necrosis, and other myopathic changes.[17] Such patients may be nonambulatory if they have significant involvement and little functional use of the lower extremities. PROM needs to be done to maintain range of motion. Patients are clearly unable to use these extremities for aerobic exercises or strengthening programs.[36]

The hypotheses on which this classification and its exercise recommendations are based are many. First of all, it is assumed that those with less affected muscles (Classes II and III) will demonstrate many of the physiological changes seen in normal muscle as described earlier. Second, as people get older, some of the motor learning adaptations that De Vries and Grimby discuss can also play a role in exercise training, thus counterbalancing the effects of motor unit dropout. Again, this is seen in the Class II and III muscles. However, when new weakness develops (Class IV) there is usually an indication of overuse, unless that extremity has been immobilized for a period of time, in which case a component of disuse is possible. Last, although difficult to prove, it is possible that many of the symptoms that individuals with post-polios develop—in particular, fatigue—are due to deconditioning, as many studies have shown that with conditioning, people are able to perform routine tasks with less fatigue. Though these recommendations have been used successfully in our clinic, and the literature in part supports this, we acknowledge that only through further prospective studies that use these criteria as well as quantitative measurements will the development of more specific guidelines be possible.

CONCLUSION

It has been demonstrated that people with a history of polio can improve muscular strength and endurance as well as cardiovascular conditioning by way of an exercise program. With this in mind and using the limb-specific classification system described earlier, an appropriately trained professional can develop a prescription for a rational exercise program so that post-polio individuals can more safely enjoy many of the additional positive benefits that regular exercise can bring.

REFERENCES

1. Agre JC: Quantification of neuromuscular function in post-polio subjects and the effects of muscle strengthening exercises. Presented at the AAPM&R course "Future role of muscular strengthening exercises in the rehabilitatory management of patients with neuromuscular disorders," November 1992.

2. Agre JC, Rodriguez AA: Intermittent isometric activity: Its effect on muscle fatigue in post-polio patients. Arch Phys Med Rehabil 72:971–975, 1991.

3. Agre JC, Rodriguez AA: Neuromuscular function: Comparison of symptomatic and asymptomatic polio subjects to control subjects. Arch Phys Med Rehabil 71:545–551, 1990.

4. Agre JC, Rodriguez AA: Neuromuscular function in polio survivors at one year follow up. Arch Phys Med Rehabil 72:7–10, 1991.

5. Agre JC, Rodriguez AA: Neuromuscular function in polio survivors. Orthopedics 14:1343–1347, 1991.

6. Agre JC, Rodriguez AA, Tafel JA: Late effects of polio: Critical review of the literature on neuromuscular function. Arch Phys Med Rehabil 72:923–931, 1991.

7. Alba AA, et al: Exercise testing as a useful tool in the physiatric management of the post-polio survivor. In Halstead LS, Weichers DO (eds): Research and Clinical Aspects of the Late Effects of Poliomyelitis. Birth Defects 23(4):301–313, 1987.

8. American College of Sports Medicine: Guidelines for Exercise Testing and Prescription. Philadelphia, Lea & Febiger, 1986.

9. Beasly WC: Quantitative muscle testing principles and applications to research and clinical services. Arch Phys Med Rehabil 42:398–425, 1961.

10. Bennett RL, Knowlton GC: Overwork weakness in partially denervated muscle. Clin Orthop 12:122–49, 1958.

11. Borg GA: Perceived exertion as an indicator of somatic stress. Scand J Rehabil Med 2:92–98, 1970.

12. Borg GA: Psychosocial bases of perceived exertion. Med Sci Sports Exerc 14:377–381, 1982.

13. Borg KB, et al: Effects of excessive use of remaining muscle fibers in prior polio and LV lesion. Muscle Nerve 11:1219–1230, 1988.

14. Cashman NR, et al: Late denervation in patients with antecedent paralytic poliomyelitis. N Engl J Med 317:7–12, 1987.

15. Cashman NR, et al: Post-poliomyelitis syndrome: Evidence of ongoing denervation in symptomatic and asymptomatic patients. In Halstead LS, Weichers DO (eds): Research and Clinical Aspects of the Late Effects of Poliomyelitis. Birth Defects 23(4):237–240, 1987.

16. Codd MB, et al: Poliomyelitis in Rochester, Minnesota, 1935–1955: Epidemiology and long-term sequelae: a preliminary report. In Halstead LS, Weicher DO, eds: Late effects of Poliomyelitis. Miami, Symposia Foundation, 1985, pp 121–133.

17. Dalakas MC: Morphological changes in the muscles of patients with post-poliomyelitis neuromuscular symptoms. Neurology 38:99–104, 1988.

18. Dalakas MC: New neuromuscular symptoms in old poliomyelitis: A three year follow up study. Eur Neurol 25:381–387, 1986.

19. Dalakas MC, et al: A long term follow up study of patients with post-poliomyelitis neuromuscular symptoms. N Engl J Med 15:959–963, 1986.

20. Dean ED, Ross J: Modified aerobic walking program: Effect on patients with post-polio syndrome symptoms. Arch Phys Med Rehabil 69:1033–1038, 1988.

21. DeLateur BJ, Lehman LF: Strengthening exercise. In Leek JC, Gershwin EM, Fowler WM (eds): Principles of Physical Medicine and Rehabilitation in the Musculoskeletal Diseases. Orlando, FL, Grune & Stratton, 1986.

22. Delorme TL, Scwab RS, Watkins AL: The response of the quadriceps femoris to progressive resistance exercises in poliomyelitis patients. J Bone Joint Surg 30A:834–847, 1948.

23. Delorme TL, Watkins AL: Technics of progressive resistance exercises. Arch Phys Med 29:263–274, 1948.

24. de Vries H: Physiology of exercise for physical education and athletics. Dubuque, Iowa, William Brown Co, 1974, pp 366–376.

25. Einarsson G: Muscle conditioning in late poliomyelitis. Arch Phys Med Rehabil 72:11–14, 1991.

26. Einarsson G, Grimby G: Strengthening exercise program in post-polio subjects. In Halstead LS, Weichers DO (eds): Research and Clinical Aspects of the Late Effects of Poliomyelitis. Birth Defects 23(4):275–283, 1987.

27. Einarsson G, Grimby G, Stalberg E: Electromyographical and morphological function compensation in late poliomyelitis. Muscle Nerve 13:165–171, 1990.

28. Feldman RM: The use of strengthening exercises in post-polio sequelae. Orthopedics 8:889–890, 1985.

29. Feldman RM, Soskolne CL: The use of nonfatiguing strengthening exercises in post-polio syndrome. In Halstead LS Weichers DO, eds: Late Effects of Poliomyelitis. Miami, Symposia Foundation, 1985, pp 335–341.

30. Fillyaw MJ, et al: The effects of long-term non-fatiguing resistance exercises in subjects with post-polio syndrome. Orthopedics 14:1253–1256, 1991.

31. Gawne AC, Aseff JN, Halstead LS: Electrodiagnostic findings in patients with a history of polio. Arch Phys Med Rehabil 72:813, 1991.

32. Gawne AC, Halstead LS: Exercise in post-polio patients: A new classification. Arch Phys Med Rehabil 74:660, 1993.

33. Gawne AC, Halstead LS: Unexpected neurological findings in 66 consecutive post-polio patients. Arch Phys Med Rehabil 74:667–668, 1993.

34. Grimby G, Einarsson G: Muscle morphology with special reference to muscle strength in post-polio patients. In Halstead LS, Weichers DO (eds): Late Effects of Poliomyelitis. Miami, Symposia Foundation, 1985, pp 335–334.

35. Grimby G, et al: Muscle adaptive changes in post-poliomyelitis subjects. Scand J Rehabil Med 21:1926, 1989.

36. Gurewitsch AD: Intensive graduated exercises in early infantile paralysis. Arch Phys Med 31:213–218, 1950.

37. Halstead LS: Assessment and differential diagnosis for post-polio syndrome. Orthopedics 14:1209–1217, 1991.

37a. Halstead LS, Gawne AC, Pham BT: NRH limb-specific exercise classification for exercise, research and clinical trials in post-polio patients. In The Post-Polio Syndrome: Advances in the Pathogenesis and Treatment. Ann N Y Acad Sci 1994, in press.

38. Halstead LS, Rossi CD: New problems in old polio patients: Results of a survey of 539 polio survivors. Orthopedics 8:845–850, 1985.

39. Halstead LS, Rossi CD: Post-polio syndrome: Clinical experience with 132 consecutive of poliomyelitis. Birth Defects 23(4):13–26, 1987.

40. Halstead LS, Weichers DO (eds): Late Effects of Poliomyelitis. Miami, Symposia Foundation, 1985, pp 15–20.

41. Hettinger T, Muller EM: Muskelleisung an muskel training. Arbeitsphysiol 15:111–126, 1953.

42. Jones DR, et al: Cardiorespiratory responses to aerobic training by patients with postpoliomyelitis sequelae. JAMA 261:3255–3288, 1989.

43. Kilfoil MR, St. Pierre DM: Reliability of Cybex II isokinetic evaluations of torque in post poliomyelitis. Arch Phys Med Rehabil 74:730–735, 1993.

44. Knowlton GC, Bennett RL: Overwork. Arch Phys Med 38:18–20, 1957.

45. Kriz JL et al: Cardiorespiratory responses to upper extremity aerobic training by post-polio subjects. Arch Phys Med Rehabil 73:49–54, 1992.

46. Lange L: Uber funktionelle Anpassung, Berlin, Springer Verlag, 1919.

47. Lovett RW: The treatment of infantile paralysis. JAMA 64:2118, 1915.

48. Matthews DK, Fox EL: The Physiological Basis of Physical Education and Athletics. Philadelphia, W.B. Saunders, 1976, pp 135–149.

49. Mortini T, deVries HA: Neural factors vs hypertrophy in the time course of muscle strength gain. Am J Phys Med 58:115–130, 1979.

50. Mortini T, deVries HA: Potential for gross muscle hypertrophy in older men. J Gerontol 35:645–667, 1980.

51. Munin MC, et al: Post-poliomyelitis muscle weakness: A prospective study of quadriceps strength. Arch Phys Med Rehabil 72:729–733, 1991.

52. Munstat TL, Andres P, Thibideau L: Preliminary observations on long term muscle forces changes in the post-polio syndrome. In Halstead LS, Weichers DO (eds): Research and Clinical Aspects of the Late Effects of Poliomyelitis. Birth Defects 23(4):329–334, 1987.

53. Nelson KR: Creatinine kinase and fibrillation potentials in patients with late sequelae of polio. Muscle Nerve 13:722–755, 1990.

54. Owens RR, Jones D: Polio residuals clinic, conditioning exercise program. Orthopedics 8:882–883, 1985.

55. Perry J, Barnes G, Gronley JK: The post-polio syndrome: An overuse phenomenon. Clin Orthop 233:145–162, 1988.

56. Pollock ML, Wilmore JH: Exercise in Health and Disease: Evaluation and Prescription for Prevention and Rehabilitation. Philadelphia, W.B. Saunders, 1990, pp 202–231.

57. Ravits J, et al: Clinical and electromyographical studies of post-poliomyelitis muscular atrophy. Muscle Nerve 13:667–674, 1990.

58. Trojan DA, Gendron D, Cashman NR: Electrophysiology and electrodiagnosis of the post-poliomyelitis motor unit. Orthopedics 12:1353–1361, 1991.

59. Weichers DO: Pathophysiology and late changes of the motor unit after polio. In Halstead LS, Weichers DO (eds): Late Effects of Poliomyelitis. Miami, Symposia Foundation, 1985, pp 91–94.

60. Weichers DO: Pathophysiology and late changes in the motor unit as revealed by electromyography. Orthopedics 8:870–872, 1986.

61. Weichers DO, Hubbel SL: Late changes in the motor unit after acute polio myelitis. Muscle Nerve 4:524–528, 1981.

10

Functional Limitations and Disability in Post-Polio

GUNNAR GRIMBY, MD, PhD

Persons who have contracted polio and have remaining paresis may suffer, as is well known and described in a number of reports,[8,13,18] from different permanent and new health problems, such as fatigue, muscle weakness, muscle and joint pain, walking or other ambulation difficulties, and, in some cases, breathing problems. The concepts in the World Health Organization's (WHO) *International Classification of Impairments, Disabilities and Handicaps*[10] are used in this chapter, as is the concept of functional limitation[14], being the restrictions in basic physical and mental actions, such as ambulation, reaching, gripping, climbing stairs, and producing intelligible speech. Disability in the WHO definition refers to any restriction or inability to perform an activity in the manner or within the range considered normal for a human being when used with a specific aim. A disability often depends on several functional limitations. Personal and instrumental are the disability areas most commonly assessed in the various activities of daily living (ADL) instruments. From a broader perspective, disability also includes different aspects of social life, such as home activities, leisure activities, and work. The handicap concept, by contrast, focuses on the disadvantage for the individual, the cause being a combination of individual and environmental factors. These different levels of functional consequences of diseases or injuries are summarized in Figure 1.

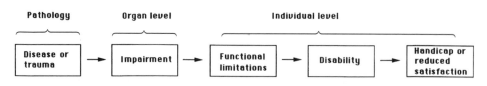

FIGURE 1. Levels of functional consequences of disease or injury.

In this chapter, the occurrence of impairments (especially with respect to muscle function), functional limitations, disabilities and resulting handicaps, and reduced quality of life in persons with poliomyelitis sequelae is reviewed, with special emphasis on the relationships between impairment, functional limitation, and disability. The use of different instruments for assessing disability is described in cross-sectional and follow-up studies in post-polio subjects. The importance of addressing disability in planning rehabilitation interventions is emphasized. The coping process, especially concerning adaptation and acceptance of new health problems with functional consequences, is discussed, as this is an important area in the management of post-polio problems.

FUNCTIONAL LIMITATION AND DISABILITY AREAS IN POST-POLIO SYNDROME

Most new symptoms in post-polio individuals relate to mobility, as paresis seems to be more common in the lower than in the upper extremities.[13,18] As most patients have no or only limited disability within personal ADL areas,[2] (e.g., dressing, bathing) it is expected that new or increased degree of disability will be within instrumental ADL areas (e.g., cleaning, washing, shopping, transportation) and often related to locomotor functions. The most common daily activities for which post-polio subjects perceived increased difficulties in a questionnaire survey were walking on level surfaces, climbing stairs, and meeting the physical demands of job and home (55–74% of the subjects).

In a recent large nationwide survey of over 3,000 polio survivors (response rate, 77%) in Denmark, Lonnberg[13] has reported new health problems in the majority of subjects: fatigue during exercise in 63%, considerable weakness in previously affected muscles in 63%, and joint pain in 51%. The prevalence of these new health problems were higher in women than in men, an observation made also in other reports.[8] The ADL problems were predominantly related to walking, with new problems in climbing stairs being most common (54%). Only around 20% had new problems related to personal ADL.

More detailed information on the occurrence of functional limitations and disabilities is given in the report by Einarsson and Grimby,[2] but in a smaller group of polio persons ($n = 41$). Seventy-one percent of these subjects met the criteria for post-polio syndrome.[8] As measured with Katz' ADL index,[12] independence in personal ADL activities was demonstrated in nearly 80% of the subjects, being the same proportion as in the larger Danish study.[13] Bathing was the most common activity with dependency. Only about half of the subjects could easily stand up from a chair. There was, as expected, a large prevalence of functional limitations in light to moderate activities, with difficulties in walking one (69%) or several blocks or climbing one flight of stairs (80%), as well as in more vigorous activities around the house or lifting heavy objects (86%) as assessed by the Functional Status Questionnaire.[11] The occurrence of ambulation disabilities is illustrated by the great problems in using public transportation, which could be used easily by only 12% of the subjects and not at all by nearly 40%. These numbers correspond to the occurrence of mobility disability in other activities noted earlier. Thirty percent of the subjects had a special handicapped transportation license, and six additional persons received a license which illustrates the need for intervention. A large number of subjects also needed assistance in household activities (spouses not counted). In the group studied, about 70% needed such assistance, and only 30% were completely independent. The type of help given usually did not involve personal ADL activities but involved activities such as cleaning or similar labor and shopping.

COMPARISON BETWEEN STABLE AND UNSTABLE POLIO SUBJECTS

In the studies described here, persons with polio were not divided into those with and without new symptoms. As new or increased muscle weakness is a common new complaint, comparison of functional limitation, disability, handicap, and health-related quality of life was made in subjects with polio acknowledging (unstable) and not acknowledging (stable) new or increased muscle weakness. Data from a 4–5 year follow-up reported by Grimby and Thorén-Jönsson[7] illustrate further differences in the development of disability and handicap according to the WHO classification between unstable and stable subjects.

STUDY GROUP

Fifty-nine persons aged 31–70 years with polio infection 29–66 years previously were studied. Thirty-four of the subjects belonged to the groups described previously by Einarsson and Grimby[2] and had various degrees of disability. Twenty-five of the subjects belonged to a group studied by Ernstoff et al.,[3] for which the selection criterion was the ability to walk with or without canes or crutches. The subjects in the first group were traced through the hospital register of patients diagnosed with polio, whereas the second group was recruited through advertisements in the newspapers and the patient organization. The patients grouped together represent a spectrum of polio patients. Fifty-five percent of the subjects met the criteria of post-polio syndrome. Sixty-six percent were categorized as unstable (new or increased weakness before or during the follow-up period) or had severe bilateral muscle atrophy (no strength measurements available). Those subjects who did not report new muscle weakness or no muscle weakness at all in their polio-affected muscles were labeled stable.

METHODS

Patients were interviewed concerning polio history, clinical symptoms related to polio, and other health problems. Muscle strength was measured with a Cybex or Kin-Com dynamometer for knee extension and knee flexion, for isometric contraction at 60° knee angle, and for isokinetic concentric and eccentric actions at various velocities.[4]

Katz' ADL index[12] for personal ADL activities, the Functional Status Questionnaire (FSQ)[11] for personal and instrumental ADL activities and problems related to mental health and social situations, and the WHO handicap classification from the *International Classification of Impairments, Disabilities and Handicaps* (ICIDH)[10] were used. The Nottingham Health Profile[9] was used as an instrument of "health-related quality of life." A summary of the content of these different instruments is given in Table 1. For the follow-up, data are only available from some of the instruments.

Statistical analyses were made with nonparametric analyses (Mann-Whitney) for both group and individual comparisons.

RESULTS

Cross-Sectional Data

Presentation of results is first given for the group as a whole, with comparison between unstable and stable subjects.

Difficulty in personal ADL activities was uncommon (10%) and oc-

Table 1. Summary of the Content of the Assessment Instruments

	No. Items	Domains	No. of Grading Alternatives	Type of Assessment	Administration
Katz ADL	6	Personal ADL	2	Dependency	Observer
Functional Status Questionnaire (FSQ)	34 (+6 single items)	Personal and instrumental ADL Well-being Social activity and interaction Work	4 or 6	Degree of difficulty or rate of occurrence of problems	Self-assessment
WHO Handicap Classification	5 (6)	Orientation Mobility Physical independence Occupation Social interaction (economy not used)	8	Degree of involvement	Observer
Nottingham Health Profile	45	Energy, physical mobility, pain, sleep, emotional reactions, social isolation Different life areas	2	Affirmation of statements	Self-assessment

curred only in subjects with new weakness (*see also* data from FSQ in Table 2). Instrumental ADL (mobility) was more affected, whereas mental health and social interaction were rather moderately impaired. Eighty percent of the subjects were working, and the scores for work were moderately reduced in some of these persons, implying limited working hours, adaptation of the working place, or various limitations in working ability and performance. The unstable subjects had significantly lower scores than the stable subjects for all FSQ scales except mental health and quality of social interaction (Table 2).

The classification of handicap according to the WHO demonstrated an usually low degree of handicap in orientation, physical dependence, and social interaction (median values 1, 0, and 2, respectively) but a higher degree of handicap in mobility (median value 3). The unstable subjects had a significantly higher degree of handicap for mobility, occupation, and social integration than the stable subjects (Table 2).

Table 2. Comparison Between Stable and Unstable Polio Subjects

	Stable (n = 20)		Unstable (n = 39)		
	Median	Range	Median	Range	*p* Value
FSQ score*					
Basal ADL	100	9–100	89	0–100	<0.001
Instrumental ADL	76	24–100	45	19–95	<0.001
Mental health	84	52–100	80	48–100	ns
Social activity	100	44–100	78	11–100	<0.05
Quality of social interaction	86	56–100	92	48–100	ns
Work†	100	83–100	88	17–100	<0.001
WHO handicap‡					
Orientation	1	0–1	1	0–3	ns
Physical independence	0	0–4	0	0–7	ns
Mobility	0	0–5	3	0–5	<0.001
Occupation	0	0–5	4	0–7	<0.001
Social integration	0	0–3	2	0–6	<0.01
Nottingham Health Profile⁶					
Energy	0	0–63	24	0–100	<0.01
Physical mobility	0	0–72	38	0–100	<0.001
Pain	0	0–48	19	0–82	<0.001
Sleep	0	0–75	16	0–88	ns
Emotional reactions	0	0–68	8	0–60	<0.05
Social isolation	0	0–64	0	0–25	ns

*For FSQ, 0 is most affected, 100 is unaffected.
†Number of both stable and unstable subjects was 18.
‡WHO handicap classification, 0 is no handicap, 8 is highest handicap level.
§For the Nottingham Health Profile 0 is unaffected, 100 is maximal affected (ns = not significant).

The Nottingham Health Profile showed no or only moderate distress in the various dimensions, with a median value being above 0 only for physical mobility (30 of a maximum of 100 being most affected), but with large individual variations. The unstable subjects had lower scores than the stable subjects for energy, physical mobility, pain, and emotional reactions (Table 2). Problems with different areas in daily life were identified with the Profile's part II and also found to be more frequent in the unstable than in the stable group concerning household activities, social contacts, leisure time activities, and holidays; thus all areas were affected except family life (Table 3).

Muscle strength for isometric knee extension at 60° knee angle was

Table 3. Subjects with Problems in Areas Assessed by the Nottingham Health Profile Part II

	Stable (n = 20)	Unstable (n = 34)	p Value
Household activities	4	24	<0.01
Social contacts	1	14	<0.05
Family life	0	6	ns
Leisure activities	1	16	<0.05
Holidays	5	21	<0.05

ns = not significant.

60% (SD 25) of predicted normal values in 20 measured stable subjects and 34% (SD 20) in 25 measured unstable subjects ($p<0.001$) The corresponding values for isokinetic knee extension at 60°/s angular velocity were 63% (SD 27) and 36% (SD 21) for the stable and unstable groups, respectively ($p<0.01$). Thus, the group acknowledging new or increased weakness (unstable) also showed objective evidence of lower muscle strength values than the stable group.

Four–Five-Year Follow-Up

During the follow-up period, muscle strength (concentric knee extension with an angular velocity of 60°/s) decreased in 44 measured subjects an average of 9% ($p<0.01$) and from 53 to 48% of control values. Similar reductions were found in other measures of knee extension strength. When the subjects were divided into stable and unstable, the unstable group but not the stable group showed a significant reduction in strength (5% and 16%, respectively). Thus, the perception of further reduction in muscle strength could be verified objectively by dynamometer measurements.

Only 2 new subjects (out of 59) developed dependence in personal ADL. As an example of the increase in mobility limitations, the number of wheelchair users increased from 7 at the first examination to 13 at the second examination. In addition, public transportation was more difficult to use at the second than at the first examination. Thirty-seven percent of the subjects had problems with this activity at the first examination, compared to 49% at the second examination.

All the handicap categories according to the WHO classification showed a small but significant increase ($p<0.05$–0.01) during the follow-up period. However, when the patients were divided into those with and without new or increased symptoms, it was only the former group who showed a significant ($p<0.05$–0.001) increase in the degree of handicap.

GENERAL DISCUSSION

There may be several explanations for the new health problems (e.g. increased fatigue, new or increased muscle weakness, pain in muscle and joints, and breathing problems) in post-polio subjects, as discussed in various chapters of this volume. It is difficult from the information available to analyze in any detail the relationships between impairments, functional limitations, and disabilities leading to different levels of handicap. Disabilities in this group of patients are, however, often related to mobility performance, lower extremity muscles being more commonly affected.[13,18] Muscle function therefore, was specially studied, and for purposes of analysis, the polio subjects were divided into stable (no new weakness) and unstable (new or increased weakness, including already severe muscle atrophy) groups. The reasons for the reduction in muscle strength and function may be several (*see* chapter 2 by Stålberg and Grimby). There are clear indications of an ongoing remodeling process in the polio-affected muscles, with denervation-reinnervation and changes in the size of muscle fibers[1,6] leading to reduction in muscle function in some individuals. The muscle strength may also be secondarily reduced as a consequence of reduced physical activity, which, in turn, can be due to reduced muscle strength and endurance, general fatigue from other reasons, or pain; thus, the polio subject develops a vicious circle leading to increasing degrees of disability.

All changes on the impairment level, even with new functional limitations, may not lead to reduction in ability to perform various activities in daily living (disability level) and to handicap. In the group of polio subjects studied in our department, changes were recorded in disabilities during the follow-up period, but to a limited extent. The degree of handicap according to the WHO classification, although generally low, increased for all categories. It is of interest to note that the increase was significant for those patients perceiving new or increased muscle weakness, but not for those without such a report, indicating the significance of clinical symptoms and decline of functions for a reduced ability in various areas of daily life.

Increased impairment and functional limitations may lead to a perceived increase in disability, but only to a certain extent. Function has to be reduced beyond a certain threshold level until the ability for a certain activity is reduced. Furthermore, the strategy to try to surpass the limit of one's capacity and to minimize the perception of new difficulties[7] makes the relationship among impairment, disability, and handicap difficult to determine. The relationship between impairment or functional limitation and ability to perform various activities needing that type of function is hypothetically suggested to be stepwise. Function has to be reduced by a certain new amount before the ability to perform a specific task is abolished, although an increasing degree of difficulty may have been perceived earlier. In this group of patients, this can, however, often be neglected. At a certain threshold level, the ability for a specific activity is abolished, or in the opposite direction, a certain functional level must be reached (e.g., a minimal muscle strength or joint mobility) to allow for a defined activity (e.g., stair-climbing). The relationship between function and ability for a certain activity can also be changed by successive modifications of the environment, e.g., new or more frequent use of walking aids to get around, or handrails and supporting rails in the bathroom. Thus, independence may be maintained despite an increased degree of impairment and functional limitations.

The post-polio situation is a typical example of secondary impairments, such as a new muscle weakness and fatigue, leading to secondary disabilities[15,19] on top of the original disabilities. There is a need for multidisciplinary support, as these new conditions will interfere with most life areas. Due to the previous coping strategies to "fight" functional limitations, the polio persons themselves may not observe or accept the consequences of their reduced function and are therefore less ready to try to find new strategies and solutions.[7] As a result, some of them may perceive unspecified anxiety and reduced well-being. It is important to remember, however, that coping with the new health problems and adapting the environment more appropriately are dynamic processes. The impact on well-being, health-related quality of life, and degree of handicap reported in cross-sectional studies should therefore be looked upon as time-limited samples of information.

Comparing stable and unstable polio subjects, it is important to note that the impact of new weakness is more marked in the unstable subjects, not only on dimensions related to physical function but also and to a lesser degree on social-related dimensions (with the exception of family life). The impact on mental health is, however, in general low and does not differ significantly between these two groups of subjects. Thus, despite what is examplified and discussed concerning coping problems and risks for reduced well-being, the post-polio subject in general does not report much increased distress in mental and emotional areas.

The different instruments used in our studies should be regarded only as examples that illustrate the possibility of combining findings of changes in function, dependence and difficulties in daily activities, well-being, and health-related quality of life to depict a broad description of patient problems. As most problems are outside the personal ADL in the majority of polio subjects, the Katz ADL index does not usually provide much information. The FSQ describes the perceived difficulties in various areas and can be used as a screening instrument. In addition, it provides data on mental health and social interaction. The WHO handicap classification is not an instrument but rather a taxonomy, and it has conceptual problems with some of the categories (e.g., physical independence and mobility are not clearly distinguishable from disability). In contrast to the FSQ and Nottingham Health Profile, the grading is made by the observer. The Nottingham Health Profile is a short instrument dealing with "health-related quality of life" and demonstrates differences in impact on various dimensions between subjects with and without new symptoms. It can probably be useful in further follow-up studies. Other instruments describing the degree of dependence not only in personal but also in instrumental ADL activities are available, and the reader is referred for a review to a recent book by Wade.[17]

The importance of a broad approach in cross-sectional as well as follow-up studies in chronic conditions with secondary disabilities should be stressed. The methods may be chosen according to the previous experience of the investigator or clinician and depending on the patient population. In clinical work, a thorough and individually chosen analysis should be made of the disability situation of the patient, including environmental-dependent aspects, even if the treatment approach is mainly on the impairment level. By not addressing the disability area primarily, the clinician may limit the intervention to the impairment or functional limitation areas, e.g., mobility training in a patient with major stair-climbing difficulties. However, there will be no major impact on the disability situation until the need for stair-climbing has been abolished. The goals of the patient and his or her coping strategy and capacity should also always be an important part of the intervention planning.

ACKNOWLEDGMENTS

The author thanks Professor Alan Jette at the New England Research Institute, Watertown, Massachusetts, for valuable advice, especially concerning the Functional Status Questionnaire. The studies were supported by grants from King Gustav V's 80 Years Foundation, the Medical Research Council (Proj. 03888), the Research Council of Social Science, and the National Association of the Traffic Accident and Polio Disabled.

REFERENCES

1. Einarsson G, Grimby G, Stålberg E: Electromygraphic and morphological functional compensation in late poliomyelitis. Muscle Nerve 13:165–171, 1991.

2. Einarsson G, Grimby G: Disability and handicap in late poliomyelitis. Scand J Rehabil Med 22:113–121, 1990.

3. Ernstoff B, Wetterqvist H, Kvist H, Grimby G: The effects of endurance training on individuals with post-poliomyelitis. (In preparation.)

4. Grimby G, Einarsson G, Hedberg M, Aniansson A: Muscle adaptive changes in post-polio subjects. Scand J Rehabil Med 21:19–26, 1989.

5. Grimby G, Finnstam J, Jette A: On the application of the WHO-handicap classification in rehabilitation. Scand J Rehabil Med 20:93–98, 1988.

6. Grimby G, Stålberg E, Einarsson G: Muscle functional compensation of late polio. Arch Phys Med Rehabil 73:1000, 1992.

7. Grimby G, Thorén-Jönsson A-L: Disability in late polio. Phys Ther 74:415–424, 1994.

8. Halstead LS, Rossi CD: Post-polio syndrome: Clinical experience with 132 consecutive outpatients. In Halstead LS, Wiechers DO (eds): Research and Clinical Aspects of the Late Effects of Poliomyelitis. Birth Defects 23(4):13–16, 1987.

9. Hunt SM, McKenna SJ: A quantitative approach to perceived health status: A validation study. J Epidemiol Commun Health 34:281–286, 1980.

10. International Classification of Impairments, Disabilities and Handicaps: A Manual of Classification Relating to the Consequences of Disease. Geneva, World Health Organization, 1980.

11. Jette AM, Davies AR, Cleary PD et al: The Functional Status Questionnaire: Reliability and validity when used in primary care. J Gen Intern Med 1:143–149, 1986.

12. Katz S, Ford AB, Moskowitz RW, et al: Studies of illness in the aged: The Index of ADL: A standardized measure of biological and psychosocial function. JAMA 185:914–919, 1963.

13. Lonnberg F: Post-polio sequelae in Denmark: Presentation and results of a nationwide survey of 3 607 polio survivors. Scand J Rehabil Med Suppl 28:1–32, 1993.

14. Nagy SZ: Disability concepts revisited: Implications for prevention. In Pope AM, Tarlow AR (eds): Disability in America. Washington, D.C., National Academic Press, 1991, pp 307–327.

15. Pope AM, Tarlow AR: Prevention of secondary conditions. In Pope AM, Tarlow AR, eds: Disability in America. Washington, D.C., National Academic Press, 1991, pp 214–241.

16. Reference deleted.

17. Wade DT: Measurement in Neurological Rehabilitation. Oxford, Oxford University Press, 1992.

18. Westbrook MT: A survey of post-poliomyelitis sequelae: Manifestations, effects on people's lives and responses to treatment. Aust Physiother 37:89–102, 1991.

19. Westbrook MT, McDowell LM: Coping with a secondary disability: Implications of the late effects of poliomyelitis for occupational therapists. Aust Occup Ther J 38:83–91, 1991.

11

Psychosocial Issues and Post-Polio: A Literature Review of the Past Thirteen Years

JANET M. LIECHTY, MSW

The past decade has seen an expansion of public interest, professional literature, and research in the area of poliomyelitis and post-polio sequelae. However, this condition still presents many unanswered questions. One of the many ongoing research challenges is to describe the psychosocial issues faced by persons with a history of polio and the relationship, if any, of these variables to physical symptoms. That challenge was identified in the first symposium on post-polio held in Warm Springs, Georgia, in 1984,[45] and efforts to respond to this challenge continue today.

As inquiry into the late effects of poliomyelitis moves into its second decade, we need to evaluate the work thus far in order to describe and understand the psychosocial concerns of people with a history of polio. What do we know empirically? What do we assert we know that is actually hypothesis or overgeneralization? What gaps in knowledge exist? What questions have we tried to address with careful research? What questions do we need to address? Have the research questions been coordinated to build a knowledge base, or have the inquiries been unrelated and arbitrary? And finally, how useful has the current literature been to consumers and clinicians?

Questions such as these led to a critical review of professional literature from 1980 to 1993 that addresses the psychosocial implications of polio and post polio. The purpose of this chapter is to (a) identify and categorize psychosocial journal publications about this population; (b) summarize the major findings and assertions of these publications; (c) discuss the trends, strengths, and weaknesses of the psychosocial literature; and (d) make recommendations for future psychosocial research.

LITERATURE REVIEW METHODOLOGY

Three computerized databases were used (MEDLINE, Psychlit, and Sociofile) to conduct a search of relevant polio-related articles that appeared between 1980 and December 1993 in professional journals. Articles were deemed relevant if social, emotional, or psychological content were evident in the title or abstract and if subjects were humans with a history of polio. Exceptions were foreign-language articles, certain epidemiological studies (e.g., vaccination studies), and studies in which polio individuals made up less than 50% of an undifferentiated, general disability population.

Relevant articles were identified by searching the databases with the key words in Table 1 and by reviewing the on-line abstracts. Several additional articles were identified informally. The author was able to obtain 56 of these articles by using three local medical libraries, a university library, and an interlibrary loan service. Of the 56, 43 were deemed appropriate for this project, 11 were excluded because psychosocial content was found in less than three sentences, and 2 were excluded because the articles were strictly methodological in nature.

TABLE 1. Key Words for Database Search

Polio*	Stress
Psycholog*	Adaptation
Social	Psychosocial
Emotion*	Post-polio
Behavior*	Not immunization
Family	Not vaccine

*Indicates a search for all possible endings to given root word.

RESULTS

The 43 articles included in this review are authored by researchers in a variety of disciplines, including social workers, psychologists, physicians, nurses, physical and occupational therapists, and a seminary-degreed writer. The articles can be grouped in two main categories: research based and non-research based. The first category is subdivided according to type of research; the nonresearch category is subdivided according to the content of the articles (Table 2). This section summarizes the salient findings of the articles by category, with emphasis on the research studies and first subcategory in particular.

RESEARCH ARTICLES

Research on psychological, emotional, and behavioral aspects of polio

This subcategory consists of seven articles that reported on descriptive research with a defined methodology. The research focused on emotional, psychological, or behavioral aspects of polio as documented by standard measures, instruments, and methods. Several psychosocial domains have been investigated in the past decade. These include depression,[1,6,14,43] personality,[14,48] overall emotional and psychosocial functioning,[6] neuropsychologic functioning,[14] a type A behavioral pattern,[3] self-concept and attitudes toward other disability groups,[31] and behavioral compliance with a polio clinic's treatment recommendations.[34]

Studies of **depression** have yielded inconsistent results. Three of the studies concluded that depression scores were elevated in polio survivors; one study did not. However, comparison of each study's statistical results is restricted by several factors. These include use of different psychometric tests to measure depression, use of different cutoff criteria for depression when the same tests are used by different studies, lack of uniform presentation of statistical data, and lack of uniform definition of population groups (some included all polio survivors and some only those with post-polio symptoms). Comparing findings is further complicated by the wide variation in quality of methodological design (e.g., sample size, sampling method, validity, reliability).

Depression was found in 23% of 86 polio survivors as measured by a score greater than 14 on the Beck Depression Inventory (BDI) by Berlly et al.[1] In another study, mean BDI scores of only 11.5 for subjects with post-polio syndrome ($n = 13$) and 12.1 for polio subjects without post-polio

TABLE 2. Classification of Articles Reviewed

Research articles (*n* = 20)

Psychological, emotional, behavioral aspects of polio (*n* = 7)	Berlly et al., 1991[1] Bruno & Frick,1987[3] Conrady et al., 1989[6] Freidenberg et al., 1989[14] Nwuga, 1985[31] Peach & Olejnik, 1991[34] Tate et al., 1993[43]
Case study (*n* = 1)	Hammond, 1991[22]
Ethnographic (sociocultural, historical, political, biographical) (*n* = 4)	Fischer, 1989[10] Kaufert & Locker, 1990[24] Locker et al, 1987[28] Scheer & Luborsky, 1991[36]
Epidemiologic, social, demographic (*n* = 8)	Einarrson & Grimby, 1990[9] Foster et al., 1993[12] Halstead et al., 1985[21] Owen, 1985[32] Shaar & McCarthy, 1992[37] Speier et al., 1987[40] Windebank et al., 1987[47] Windebank et al., 1991[48]

Nonresearch articles (*n* = 23)

Clinical observations or impressions (*n* = 7)	Bruno & Frick, 1991[2] Bruno et al., 1991[4] Freedman, 1981[13] Frick, 1985[15] Frick & Bruno, 1986[16] Kohl, 1987[26] Maynard & Roller, 1991[29]
Testimonials (*n* = 4)	Byrne et al., 1982[5] Heisler, 1984[23] Post-polio Network, 1991[35] Smith, 1989[39]
Rehabilitation overviews (*n* = 10)	Currie et al.,1993[7] Dean, 1991[8] Frustace, 1988[17] Halstead, 1988[20] Halstead, 1991[18] Twist & Ma, 1986[44] Williams & Douglass, 1986[46] Winters, 1991[49] Young, 1989[51] Young, 1991[50]
News (*n* = 2)	Smith, 1989[38] Swan, 1984[42]

syndrome (*n* = 12) were considered moderately elevated by the authors.[14] These two groups of researchers interpreted the BDI scores differently and reported results differently, which limits meaningful comparison of the two groups' findings.

Conrady et al. found that the depression subscale scores of the Symptom Checklist 90 Revised (SCL-90R) were elevated in people with histories of polio (*n* = 93).[6] However, Tate et al. used the Brief Symptom Inventory (BSI) to assess depression and psychological distress and found that overall BSI scores among 116 polio survivors were in the normal range.[43] The Tate group also found that those subjects who demonstrated depression reported increased pain, decreased health status, decreased satisfaction with life and work, and poorer coping behaviors. In contrast, the Freidenberg et al.[14] and Conrady et al.[6] studies found that depression scores were not correlated with post-polio symptomatology or level of physical disability, respectively. These inconsistencies may be due to methodologic variances, such as whether an objective or a phenomenologic approach to symptom and distress identification within the study is employed.

Conrady et al. made a needed contribution to the understanding of depression and polio in their discussion of the difficulty of diagnosing depression independent from a medical condition.[6] Due to "multiple interactions of psychobiologic determinants," it is generally not possible to determine a causal direction between post polio and depression. In addition, clinical symptoms of depression may also be common symptoms of post polio, such as sleep disturbance[11,41] or fatigue[19,33] and may have an organic rather than psychologic etiology. Scores on psychometric tests may therefore be somewhat inflated.

Freidenberg et al. also acknowledged that the most frequently cited symptoms on the BDI related to somatic complaints,[14] which could be a result of the post-polio itself. Similarly, Berlly et al. discussed the problems in diagnosing depression in polio subjects, and they presented criteria to differentiate psychologic from biologic fatigue,[1] a symptom common to depression and post polio. The study by Tate et al. cited the percentage of the general adult population that is likely to suffer a depressive episode in their life (15–30%) and compared this to the authors' findings about incidence of depression and distress among polio survivors, which was 15.8%.[43] This type of comparison offers needed perspective on findings about polio survivors.

Personality was investigated using the Minnesota Multiphasic Personality Inventory (MMPI) by one study in this category[14] and two epidemiological studies mentioned in a later section.[47,48] The Freidenberg group found that post-polio syndrome (PPS) was not significantly associated with personality disturbances (n = 13 with PPS; n = 12 without PPS). The group noted a "trend for patients with PPS to have higher scores on the MMPI scale related to introversion and lower scores on the scale related to symptoms of hypomania," though the differences were not statistically significant. These unremarkable findings regarding an association between polio and personality disorders are consistent with those of the two Windebank studies, which are discussed in the Epidemiologic Research section.

Overall psychosocial and emotional functioning was studied by Conrady et al. using the SCL-90R and the Psychosocial Adjustment to Illness Scale—Self-Report (PAIS-SR).[6] The group's sample was taken from a clinic population (n = 71) and two support groups (n = 22). Combining both groups (n = 93), the authors found elevated SCL 90-R subscale scores on somatization, depression, and psychoticism and elevated PAIS-SR subscale scores on health care orientation, social environment, and extended family relationships. They concluded that this demonstrates significant psychological distress in their sample of subjects with a history of polio.

However, they acknowledge that the SCL 90-R subscales on somatization, depression, and psychoticism may be elevated because the subscales are sensitive to the physical symptoms of PPS, such as low back and muscle pain, low energy, and "fears that something is wrong with one's body." No comparison of data on the SCL-90R or PAIS-SR between normative controls and polio subjects was provided. As mentioned earlier, psychological distress was not correlated with severity of initial polio, number of limbs involved, or use of adaptive equipment by subjects in this study.

Freidenberg et al. investigated **neuropsychological functioning**, including attention and psychomotor speed, memory, visuospatial ability, and word list generation.[14] Their population consisted of 30 polio survivors, with and without PPS, who were seen in an outpatient polio clinic. The investigators found overall performance to be in the normal range, with no significant differences between the polio subjects with a diagnosis of PPS and those without.

Bruno and Frick explored the prevalence of **type A behaviors** among polio survivors.[3] This construct was not explicitly defined in their publication. They used a seven- or ten-item (depending on employment status) yes/no questionnaire to determine type A patterns. Their control population was taken from another study of cardiac patients who were nondisabled, employed males. They found that the type A scores were significantly higher in the polio population than in the control population. They also found that type A scores were higher in both subjects who agreed with a statement that emotional stress initiates or exacerbates their physical symptoms and subjects who reported that they experienced psychophysiologic symptoms (i.e., frequent neck/back pain or muscle spasm, anxiety, headaches, and sleep problems), muscle pain, and fatigue.

It is because this intriguing study is frequently cited in subsequent publications and used as a scientific building block for new hypotheses[2,4,22] that it is necessary to consider some of the methodologic problems of this study. Methodologic concerns include sampling, clarity of terminology, and validity of instrumentation.

The researchers acknowledge that sampling control was lost and they could not document the response rate. Like any survey, it is biased by the self-selection of respondents, and all data are based on self-report alone. Self-selection bias also occurred at a higher level of the survey, as the initial survey was mailed to self-identified clinics and support groups across the United States, in addition to which it was apparently each clinic or support group's choice whether and how to distribute the questionnaire. Even so, a response by 676 subjects is notable.

The researchers use terminology that is problematic. They claim that the psychophysiologic symptoms they selected to investigate are pathognomonic of chronic stress. This is misleading, as "pathognomonic" is a term generally reserved for a condition that is unequivocally associated with and nearly synonymous with another condition. The symptoms they cite (e.g., frequent neck and back pain, muscle spasms, headaches, sleep disturbance, anxiety) are not unequivocally associated and nearly synonymous with chronic stress. To accept their hypothesis that "persons who had poliomyelitis . . . evidence psychophysiologic symptoms pathognomonic of chronic stress" includes accepting an unsubstantiated relationship between symptoms cited and chronic stress, as well as the embedded assumption that the symptoms selected are psychophysiologic in origin. The inherent ambiguity and caution required in assigning psychologic or biologic etiology to post-polio symptoms have already been discussed.

The term and construct "type A" is not explicitly defined by the authors, so the reader must make inferences about the implied meaning of type A behavior, which may or may not concur with the authors' understanding. This construct in particular requires definition, for it has gained wide usage in the popular culture and media related to heart disease and has therefore lost most of its academic specificity.

Finally, the only standard measure used in this study was the brief type A questionnaire. No other standard measures of physical symptomatology, emotional stress, activities of daily living, or functional status were described, although data were gathered in all these areas and standard measures are available. The validity and reliability of the nonstandard instruments used were not discussed.

Nwuga looked at 22 Nigerian male polio survivors' **self-concepts and attitudes** toward seven distinct disability groups and a nondisabled group as measured by two instruments.[31] He found that polio subjects (as well as all other physically disabled subjects) showed a favorable attitude toward others with the same disability and prefer to be identified with other disabled people rather than with nondisabled people. This is surprising given the observation made in the literature that polio subjects often want to "pass" as normal.[29] However, the population Nwuga studied was Nigerian and there may be cultural differences in patterns of preferred identification. No such study has been conducted with North American polio survivors. Severity of disability was not a controlled variable in this study.

Peach and Olejnik conducted a study on the effect of **behavioral compliance** on post-polio symptom treatment outcomes.[34] They categorized patients into three groups: compliers, partial compliers, and noncompliers. Their findings are that the compliers demonstrated the best outcomes at follow-up, with improvement or resolution of physical symptoms and improved muscle function; the partial compliers showed partial improvement but not as much as the compliers; and the noncompliers showed no change or worsened symptoms and muscle function. Poor compliance was attributed to (a) failure to present the symptoms to address; (b) refusal to accept recommended orthotics or lifestyle changes; (c) perception of orthotics as failure, (d) resistance to psychosocial support; (e) obesity; or (f) factors beyond individual control, such as finances.

The results of that study suggest that behavioral compliance with treatment recommendations for post polio greatly influences symptom outcome. Unfortunately, the study does not detail how compliance rates or symptom outcomes (other than for muscle strength) were objectively measured. It is unknown if there is a relationship between psychosocial well-being and likelihood of compliance.

In summary of this subcategory, although stereotyping exists about the psychosocial characteristics of people with a history of polio (e.g., all polio survivors are traumatized by early polio experience, or they have a type A or polio personality), what we know empirically is quite modest. These studies indicate the following: (a) there may be an increased incidence of depression among polio survivors, and polio symptoms may present the way depression does; (b) there is evidence of psychological distress among a group of 93 polio survivors on standard measures, and test results may be skewed by the confounding variables of post-polio physiological symptoms; (c) there is no evidence of significant personality disturbance associated with people with post-polio symptoms; (d) polio survivors responding to a survey perceive a relationship between stress and post-polio symptoms; and (e) behavioral compliance with one clinic's treatment recommendations appears to reduce symptoms. It is beyond the scope of this chapter to reiterate the wealth of stimulating information found in this subcategory of articles, and it is hoped that curious readers will refer to the original publications.

Case Study

One research-based case study in this review involved the therapeutic use of hypnosis to treat one individual with post-polio symptoms and type A personality.[22] Hammond used four standard pretests and posttests to evaluate treatment outcomes, including measures of anxiety, anger, mood, and personal orientation (e.g., self-regard and acceptance, sensitivity to own needs and feelings). Posttest results on these and other self-report variables were all favorable, with the exception of the goal of weight reduction. Hypnotherapy for this individual was beneficial in reducing anxiety, stress, depression, insomnia, and reported joint and muscle pain. Although findings cannot be generalized from one case, this study makes an important contribution to the literature. It is the only study reviewed that evaluated the effectiveness of any psychotherapeutic intervention.

Ethnographic Research

The four publications in this category highlighted research that was sociocultural or ethnographic in nature. These articles explored issues such as the meaning of the initial or secondary disability to the individuals with polio and the impact of sociocultural factors (e.g., technologic advances) on the person's psychosocial adaptation.

Using multiple interview case studies, Scheer and Luborsky studied the cultural and biographical contexts of polio disability and found that "decisions about current disability-related issues are infused with broader concerns about personal identity and the fulfillment of personal ideals, values and expectations" and that "early life disability experiences continue to be important in later life."[36] One of the unique contributions of this article is the description of people's positive as well as negative interpretations of disability events; the study demonstrates that there is no uniform meaning that survivors ascribe to their polio experiences. The study also found that the effectiveness and appropriateness of coping patterns are in part contingent upon the cultural and historical context of the individual. A functional coping pattern in one era of a person's life may prove to be dysfunctional in another era.

The other three publications in this subcategory present research about the experiences of polio survivors who use or have used ventilator support.[10,24,28] Kaufert and Locker used epidemiological survey data as well as multiple in-depth interviews with 10 respirator-dependent polio survivors to examine the relationships across time between cultural ideologies, advances and use of technology, and consumers' adaptive strategies related to their respiratory impairments.[24] They conceptualized the polio and post-polio career as having five phases: acute, rehabilitation, relative stability, transitional, and new respiratory dependence. Experiences at each phase were and are influenced by culture, ideology, and technology.

In the acute phase, the dramatic and heroic dimensions of survival were emphasized, and the primary psychosocial issue faced by subjects was the uncertainty of degree of recovery. The second phase was influenced largely by the rehabilitation ethic of individual effort, perseverance toward goal attainment, independence from any assistive devices, and competition toward maximal recovery. This ethic fostered self-blame, frustration, and a view of respiratory technology use as a symbol of moral failure. During the phase of relative stability (usually about 10–15 years), much of the rehabilitation ethic continued. Subjects valued independence and minimal use of technological support, believing the maxim "Use it or lose it."

In the transitional phase, survivors unexpectedly began experiencing symptoms of "tiredness, a lack of energy, depression and a loss of volition." Kaufert and Locker reported that many subjects viewed their new symptoms as lack of personal motivation or effort, based on the prevailing ideology.[24] This phase compelled a change in ideology and priorities and led to more openness to technological support. Subjects' preoccupation with independence was succeeded by a concern for quality of life. Subjects' reflections about the final phase of respiratory dependence dealt with their adaptation to new technology and the costs and benefits of a relationship to a machine.

Fischer reviewed the experiences of 114 polio survivors, as well as people with other diagnoses, who are on home ventilator care.[10] Based on these reviews, he discussed the essential dynamics of successful home-based ventilator use. He highlighted the importance of the following: patient's and family's active involvement in the care plan, education and training, an interdisciplinary team approach, trained care attendants when necessary, an accessible and involved equipment vendor, and 24-hour access to resource persons.

Epidemiologic Research

The eight articles in this subcategory present epidemiological, social, or demographic research studies with findings that are related to psychosocial functioning. Only the psychosocial findings of these studies are summarized here.

Owen surveyed 188 polio survivors who attended three polio-related conferences.[32] He included "Change in life style" and "Psychosocial vocational issues" in the clinical data gathered in the study, although, unfortunately, the survey results of these variables are not reported in the article. He includes psychosocial intervention recommendations (Table 3).

Halstead et al. analyzed 201 polio survivors' responses to a survey conducted in 1983.[21] Though the emphasis was on gathering descriptive data about post-polio symptoms, some psychosocial information is also reported. Approximately 18% of respondents reported personality changes, and many commented on the difficulty of getting their physicians to (a) believe their reports of new symptoms, (b) validate their fears, and (c) not dismiss their complaints as neurotic or malingering.

Windebank et al. conducted a survey of 276 polio survivors in Olmsted County, Minnesota, and administered the MMPI to all subjects.[47] Although results of the MMPI are, unfortunately, not contained in their report, the lead author indicated in the written conference discussion notes (an addendum to the article) both that there was no relationship between MMPI scores and polio symptomatology and that the MMPI results were within normal range, with the exception of the scores achieved by subjects who had a history of psychiatric hospitalization.

A later study by Windebank et al. evaluated 50 polio subjects, including psychological testing (e.g., MMPI).[47] The authors found that psychological factors were not implicated in the development of symptoms of weakness, fatigue, or limb pain and that only three of the 50 subjects were diagnosed with or being treated for depression. Similarly, they found neither any personality differences between the 50 polio subjects and a non-polio population nor any difference in personality traits between polio subjects with and without symptomatic complaints.

Speier et al. surveyed 327 polio survivors who contracted polio in

TABLE 3. Psychosocial Treatment Recommendations Found in the Literature

1. Behavior modification to reduce type A behaviors	Bruno & Frick, 1991[2]
Behavior modification to promote compliance	Kohl, 1987[26]
2. Education	Berlly et al, 1991[1]
	Fischer, 1989[10]
	Foster et al, 1993[12]
	Peach & Olejnik, 1991[34]
3. Family involvement in treatment plan	Fischer, 1989[10]
4. Group psychotherapy	Bruno & Frick, 1991[2]
5. Hypnotherapy	Hammond, 1991[22]
6. Identification of patient strengths and personal, cultural	Scheer & Luborsky, 1991[36]
resources to enhance compliance	
7. Linkage to social and community services	Fischer, 1989[10]
	Foster et al, 1993[12]
	Owen, 1985[32]
8. Positive reinforcement of compliance	Peach & Olejnik, 1991[34]
9. Psychosocial and supportive counseling	Foster et al, 1993[12]
	Owen, 1985[32]
Psychologic assessment	Conrady et al, 1989[6]
Psychotherapy to address dysfunctional beliefs, fears, and	Bruno & Frick, 1991[2]
suppressed emotions	
10. Relaxation training	Berlly et al, 1991[1]
Stress management	Bruno & Frick, 1987[3]
	Bruno et al, 1991[4]
11. Screening for depression	Berlly et al, 1991[1]
12. Support groups	Berlly et al, 1991[1]
	Frick, 1985[15]
	Frick & Bruno, 1986[16]
	Nwuga, 1985[31]
	Peach & Olejnick, 1991[34]
	Swan, 1984[42]
13. Teaching of effective coping behaviors	Tate et al, 1993[43]
14. Therapeutic recreation	Owen, 1985[32]
15. Vocational rehabilitation and assistance with disability claims	Owen, 1985[32]
16. Weight-loss structured programs or nutritional counseling	Peach & Olejnik, 1991[34]

1952 and were hospitalized in a Minneapolis facility.[40] Their study showed that 62% of the subjects graduated from high school and 29% completed one or more years of college. Employment rates were also high: 92% of subjects were employed since contracting polio (97% of males and 84% of females), and the employed subjects ranged from age to 34 to 79 years old.

Einarsson and Grimby studied 41 polio survivors.[9] Among other measures, they included a Functional Status Questionnaire (FSQ), which recorded subjects' feelings of well-being. Although the FSQ well-being item scores were not compared with a control group, the data presented suggest minimal or no disturbances.

Shaar and McCarthy conducted a study in war-plagued Lebanon of 240 polio subjects and 234 age- and sex-matched nondisabled siblings to illustrate the social consequences (degree of handicap) of functional limitations due to impairment (disability), with the matched siblings as controls.[37] The study compared each disabled and nondisabled sibling's status in the domains of education, work, social class, income, marital status, housing conditions, and mental well-being. The authors found significant differences between subjects and sibling controls in the areas of employment, social class, income, marital status, and housing conditions.

Compared to their siblings, most of the polio survivors were still residing with their family in crowded housing. However, the psychological distress among the polio population was not significantly greater than among their nondisabled siblings. Marital status disadvantage was related to lower income and female gender, but disabled women were not more likely to be disadvantaged in areas such as work and income level. Severity of disability did not determine degree of handicap (i.e., social disadvantage), and family resources (e.g., higher parental social status or income) helped to mitigate the social disadvantages subsequent to disability.

Foster et al. analyzed the survey responses of 237 polio subjects living in Maine to assess the incidence of PPS, coping status, knowledge of one's own condition, perceived need for social and health care services, and accessibility to these services.[12] A majority of subjects (55%) reported that they had no access to physicians knowledgeable about post polio; 51–60% reported no access to a variety of other related social and health care services. Polio subjects experiencing late effects were more knowledgeable about their condition, more likely to have access to needed health care services, and more likely to report coping difficulties. Perceived need for a post-polio clinic was related to being younger than age 65, employed, female, having coping difficulties, and experiencing late effects of polio.

NONRESEARCH ARTICLES

Clinical Observations and Impressions

The seven articles in this subcategory contain psychosocial content that is based on clinical observations, impressions, or hypothesis. The research methodology that was employed to support psychosocial assertions was either not presented or not explicit.

Based on their clinical observations, Maynard and Roller identify three coping patterns among polio survivors that correlate with the initial level of polio disability: Passers (people with invisible disabilities), Minimizers (people with a moderate disability), and Identifiers (severely disabled individuals).[29] They discuss the difficulty of transitioning from one coping style to the next when new polio symptoms increase the visibility of one's disability. This model of coping patterns has not yet been empirically tested and reported in the literature.

Frick and Bruno present their impressions about the psychological trauma and devastation associated with post-polio symptoms and second disability.[15,16] They also propose a stage theory of acceptance of second disability: (a) mourning, (b) downplaying physique, (c) enlarging one's scope of values, and (d) upholding asset evaluation. This model of adaptation to polio as a second disability has not yet been empirically tested and reported in the literature.

Kohl and Freedman observed a desire for cure among polio survivors—an expectation that knowledge or new technology should result in recovery, not merely improved quality of life.[13,26] Kohl considers the impact of personality styles and coping patterns on compliance. Physiological symptoms were observed to result in family and marital stress, and Kohl observes that many polio survivors are reluctant to accept new equipment or orthotics. Kohl also reviews outdated practices held by some polio survivors, such as increasing physical activity to deal with fatigue or focusing on increased strength as the primary goal of treatment.

Bruno et al. used data from pre-1950 autopsy and histopathology reports of poliomyelitis subjects, observations from the magnetic resonance imaging results of 12 polio survivors, and outcomes of a 1990 polio survey to make hypotheses about the relationship between emotional stress and certain polio symptoms.[4] They make the argument that emotional stress can induce post-polio fatigue and muscle weakness. These hypotheses require further careful study.

Testimonial Articles

Testimonial articles are those written by polio survivors or professionals working with survivors. Their authors describe personal experiences, feelings, thoughts, stages of adaptation, or the impact of early polio experience.

Smith, a polio survivor and nurse, states that her condition challenged her self-esteem and sent her through stages of shock and denial.[39] She describes flashbacks to painful earlier polio experiences during her adult post-polio clinic evaluation, initially viewing assistive aids as a sign of defeat. One of her primary adaptive strategies was to capitalize on her nursing background and knowledge to learn all she could about post polio. Smith also heralds the importance of support groups and networks.

Another account by a polio survivor describes frustration with the medical establishment and decreased self-esteem.[35] He writes that what he needed from health care professionals was understanding, practical guidance, and reassurance; instead, he was given psychotropic medications.

Heisler writes an almost poetic account of her initial polio experience.[23] She writes, "This was a bitter pill for a nine-year-old child to swallow and accept. The same moment in which I most completely experienced my powerlessness gave birth to my inner strength." She describes how she has integrated her disability into her self-concept, has used the experience for personal growth, and celebrates her gifts now as a "wounded healer."

Rehabilitation Overviews

The ten articles in this subcategory are written by rehabilitation professionals other than mental health practitioners and include some psychosocial content. New psychosocial content is not presented, but rather, existing literature is cited. Four of the articles are medical overviews; two are written from the perspective of occupational therapy, two from physical therapy, and two from nursing. The articles contain a theme of the need for professionals to understand and empathize with polio patients.

News Articles

The two articles in this category are informative, brief reports on post-polio symptoms, polio support groups, polio clinics, and other community services. They are among the countless other media reports on post polio that are not reflected neither in professional databases nor in this review. These news articles are a part of the trend to educate the public and those in the health care field about issues facing the polio population and about the range and availability of needed health care services.

DISCUSSION

The present review of more than a decade's worth of published literature on the psychosocial aspects of polio reveals an evolutionary trend. Naturally, the early psychosocial literature on polio consisted mostly of nonresearch articles such as preliminary impressions and anecdotal accounts, whereas the research articles tend to be more recent. Interestingly, many continue to cite the older psychosocial articles that were based on early impressions and assumptions rather than to cite more recent articles based on research outcomes. Perhaps this is because the early, subjective articles are emotionally engaging, which may appeal to the professional wanting to promote empathy for the polio survivors' experience. The problem is that the experiences described in anecdotal and impressionistic accounts are not necessarily factual or universal, and we may do consumers a disservice by assuming universality and sameness among them.

Though only one article studied the efficacy of a mode of psychosocial intervention (i.e., hypnosis),[22] numerous articles offered psychosocial treatment recommendations based on their research, impressions, or clinical experience (Table 3). Clearly, more evaluation studies are needed to determine which psychosocial interventions are effective and useful to consumers. For example, one way to test the hypothesis that stress induces or exacerbates post-polio symptoms (a cause-and-effect relationship that has not yet been proved or disproved) is to study the efficacy of stress management interventions.

A wide range of disciplines, each with a particular methodology or clinical focus, have been represented in this review. Researchers interested in psychosocial issues include mental health professionals, anthropologists, respiratory specialists, and epidemiologists. Such diversity exposes the field to the many different ways of identifying, organizing, naming, and interpreting human experience, but it also carries a caveat: it can be difficult to translate findings from one discipline or methodology to another, thereby impeding the collective goal of building a solid, common knowledge base. Therefore continued efforts to communicate across disciplines and methodologies can only enhance the depth of our understanding.

Epidemiologic and large-scale sociological studies can make a significant contribution to the understanding of psychosocial issues to the extent that they include, expand upon, and report on psychosocial areas of investigation. Such studies tend to have superior sampling methods, sizes, and overall research designs, which can advance the quality of psychosocial research immensely when such research questions are included in large-scale epidemiological studies.

Though depression has been the pathology most studied among polio survivors, we still have only limited knowledge about polio and depression. This understanding is confounded by the difficulty in differentiating psychologic symptoms of depression from biologic symptoms of post polio in the area of somatic complaints (e.g., fatigue and sleep disorders). At this time, the clinical usefulness of the studies serves basically to tell us that depression is a risk factor to be monitored. In addition to investigating areas of psychopathology, we need to learn more about patient strengths, adaptive coping patterns, and effective lifestyle modification efforts. If we look only for psychopathology, we will find it.

Other research areas that may be useful to consumers and practitioners include compliance enhancement studies, evaluation studies of treatment modalities (e.g., counseling, education, behavior modification, hypnosis, biofeedback, family counseling, support groups), psychosocial issues in the workplace, effective strategies for promoting accessibility in the workplace, and marital and family adaptation to disability.

Kaufert and Kaufert discussed methodological issues in a study of the long-term impact of disability and highlighted several typical design limitations.[25] These include cross-sectional designs (a limitation also cited by Tate et al.[43]) that cannot account for the dynamic nature of a chronic illness over time, sampling bias, unidimensional research, and designs that ignore the cultural context of the individual and the individual's perspective and meaning assigned to events.

Halstead called attention to the limitations of self-report questionnaires often used with polio subjects, as they may not be representative of all polio survivors, and to the lack of verification of accuracy or cause of reported symptoms.[18] Other polio researchers call for longitudinal studies,[14] larger sample sizes and cohort designs,[43] and multidimensional research that considers the interrelatedness of personality, coping, and social support variables.[6]

Kopp and Krakow discuss the importance of timing in any research on psychosocial adaptation, noting that people are more distressed and perform more poorly the closer they are to the onset of the stressor.[27] Similarly, in an early study of children with polio, Meyer observed a gradual lessening of distress and testing difficulties as time passed on from the acute polio event.[30] For our purposes, the length of time between onset of new symptoms and psychometric and psychosocial testing may be a performance variable, particularly because most studies use a clinic population that consists largely of people seeking help for new problems.

Most of the articles focusing on psychosocial factors were based on studies of individuals already experiencing post-polio symptoms rather than on the broader polio survivor population. There is no psychosocial research on either that envied 30–50% of the population who do *not* exhibit post-polio symptoms or on psychosocial factors associated with these survivors apparently resilient to the late effects of polio.

Finally, an ongoing question is whether or not researchers should view polio as a unique psychosocial entity or as a window into psychosocial adjustment to long-term disability, to aging with a disability, or to secondary disability. More cross-fertilization with other disability research may prove useful to polio survivors and also clear a path for polio research to be in a position to contribute to the larger disability and chronic illness knowledge base.

The scope of this literature review is limited, and thus many areas of discussion have necessarily been omitted. An in-depth critical review of the methodology of the psychosocial research thus far would be invaluable in order to improve the quality of future research, to assist readers in weighing the validity of study outcomes, and to catalog the reliable and valid instruments used to document difficult-to-measure variables such as functional status, fatigue, pain, and depression.

Also omitted have been (a) comparison of the polio psychosocial literature to that of the larger disability and chronic illness literature, which is profuse; (b) interpretive comparison and synthesis of findings across disciplines and methodologies; and (c) mention of international, non-English contributions to the psychosocial literature base.

CONCLUSION

As the psychosocial literature on polio matures, we hope to see more research published and with increasingly rigorous and careful methodology. We should also see a concomitant, gradual shift in professionals' understanding and assumptions about people with polio histories that reflect the new learning. Out of respect for consumers and for accuracy, we hope to refrain from unsubstantiated stereotyping, assuming universal emotional trauma and psychopathology are present, and defining individuals' experiences for them before they describe such experiences to us.

As practioners and researchers, we must demonstrate a commitment to research, rigorous methodology, and cautious conclusions. Self-referencing is a problem in a field with relatively few active researchers, and we need more researchers and practitioners to publish. In researching a psychosocial issue that has already been investigated, investigators must present data in a way that can be meaningfully compared to previous findings.

Finally, researchers need to continue to be their own best critics (as most indeed are) and be clear about the limitations of their studies, about any confounding variables, and about the need for cautious interpretation of psychosocial results. Intellectual integrity and modesty, together with a commitment to communicate and collaborate across disciplines in psychosocial research will lead us to a solid and enhanced, research-based understanding of the issues facing people with histories of polio, as well as to an honest partnership with consumers that can hopefully contribute to those consumers' health and well-being.

REFERENCES

1. Berlly MH, Strauser WW, Hall KM, et al: Fatigue in postpolio syndrome. Arch Phys Med Rehabil 72:115–118, 1991.

2. Bruno RL, Frick NM: The psychology of polio as prelude to post-polio sequelae: Behavior modification and psychotherapy. Orthopedics 14:1185–1193, 1991.

3. Bruno RL, Frick NM: Stress and "type A" behavior as precipitants of post-polio sequelae: The Felician/Columbian survey. In Halstead LS, Wiechers DO (eds): Research and Clinical Aspects of the Late Effects of Poliomyelitis. Birth Defects 23(4):145–155, 1987.

4. Bruno RL, Frick NM, Cohen J: Polioencephalitis, stress, and the etiology of post-polio sequelae. Orthopedics 14:1269–1276, 1991.

5. Byrne KM, Lattanzi SM, Morrissey M: Don't let me fall. Am J Nurs 82:1242–1245, 1982.

6. Conrady LJ, Wish JR, Agre JC, et al: Psychologic characteristics of polio survivors: A preliminary report. Arch Phys Med Rehabil 70:458–463, 1989.

7. Currie DM, Gershkoff AM, Cifu DX: Geriatric rehabilitation. 3. Mid- and late-life effects of early-life disabilities. Arch Phys Med Rehabil 74:S-413–S-416, 1993.

8. Dean E: Clinical decision making in the management of the late sequelae of poliomyelitis. Phys Ther 71:752–761, 1991.

9. Einarsson G, Grimby G: Disability and handicap in late poliomyelitis. Scand J Rehabil Med 22:113–121, 1990.

10. Fischer DA: Long-term management of the ventilator-dependent patient: Levels of disability and resocialization. Eur Respir J 2(Suppl 7):651s–654s, 1989.

11. Fischer DA: Sleep-disordered breathing as a late effect of poliomyelitis. In Halstead LS, Wiechers DO (eds): Research and Clinical Aspects of the Late Effects of Poliomyelitis. Birth Defects 23(4):115–120, 1987.

12. Foster LW, Berkman B, Wellen M, et al: Postpolio survivors: Needs for and access to social and health care services. Health Soc Work 18:139–148, 1993.

13. Freedman A: Psychopathological effects of restoring health in patients with chronic disease. Del Med J 53:495–501, 1981.

14. Freidenberg DL, Freeman D, Huber SJ, et al: Postpoliomyelitis syndrome: Assessment of behavioral features. Neuropsychiatry Neuropsychol Behav Neurol 2:272–281, 1989.

15. Frick NM: Post-polio sequelae and the psychology of second disability. Orthopedics 8:851–853, 1985.

16. Frick NM, Bruno RL: Post-polio sequelae: Physiological and psychological overview. Rehabil Lit 47:106–111, 1986.

17. Frustace SJ: Poliomyelitis: Late and unusual sequelae. Am J Phys Med Rehabil 66: 328–337, 1988.

18. Halstead LS: Assessment and differential diagnosis for post-polio syndrome. Orthopedics 14:1209–1217, 1991.

19. Halstead LS: Clinical experience with 132 consecutive outpatients. In Halstead

LS, Wiechers DO (eds): Research and Clinical Aspects of the Late Effects of Poliomyelitis. Birth Defects 23(4):13–26, 1987.

20. Halstead LS: The residual of polio in the aged. Top Geriatr Rehabil 3:9–26, 1988.

21. Halstead LS, Wiechers DO, Rossi CD: Late effects of poliomyelitis: A national survey. In Halstead LS, Wiechers DO, eds: Late Effects of Poliomyelitis. Miami, Symposia Foundation, 1985, pp 11–31.

22. Hammond DC: Hypnosis for postpolio syndrome and type-A behavior. Am J Clin Hypn 34:38–45, 1991.

23. Heisler V: I have walked in the shoes of the shaman. Psychol Perspect 15:65–70, 1984.

24. Kaufert JM, Locker D: Rehabilitation ideology and respiratory support technology. Soc Sci Med 30:867–877, 1990.

25. Kaufert PL, Kaufert JM: Methodological and conceptual issues in measuring the long term impact of disability: The experience of poliomyelitis patients in Manitoba. Soc Sci Med 19:609–618, 1984.

26. Kohl SJ: Emotional responses to the late effects of poliomyelitis. In Halstead LS, Wiechers DO (eds): Research and Clinical Aspects of the Late Effects of Poliomyelitis. Birth Defects 23(4):135–143, 1987.

27. Kopp CB, Krakow JB: The developmentalist and the study of biological risk: A view of the past with an eye toward the future. Child Dev 54:1086–1108, 1983.

28. Locker D, Kaufert JM, Kirk B: The impact of life support technology upon psychosocial adaptation to the late effects of poliomyelitis. In Halstead LS, Wiechers DO (eds): Research and Clinical Aspects of the Late Effects of Poliomyelitis. Birth Defects 23(4):157–171, 1987.

29. Maynard FM, Roller S: Recognizing typical coping styles of polio survivors can improve re-rehabilitation. Am J Phys Med Rehabil 70:70–72, 1991.

30. Meyer E: Psychological considerations in a group of children with poliomyelitis. J Pediatr 31:34–48, 1947.

31. Nwuga VC: A study of group–self identification among the disabled in Nigeria: A case for support groups. Int J Rehabil Res 8:61–67, 1985.

32. Owen RR: Polio residuals clinic and exercise protocol: Research implications. In Halstead LS, Wiechers DO (eds): Late Effects of Poliomyelitis. Miami, Symposia Foundation, 1985, pp 207–219.

33. Packer TL, Martins I, Krefting L, et al: Activity and post-polio fatigue. Orthopedics 14:1223–1226, 1991.

34. Peach PE, Olejnik S: Effect of treatment and noncompliance on post-polio sequelae. Orthopedics 14:1199–1203, 1991.

35. Post-polio Network: The late effects of polio. Med J Aust 155:393–394, 1991.

36. Scheer J, Luborsky ML: The cultural context of polio biographies. Orthopedics 14:1173–1181, 1991.

37. Shaar KH, McCarthy M: Disadvantage as a measure of handicap: A paired sibling study of disabled adults in Lebanon. Int J Epidemiol 21:101–107, 1992.

38. Smith DW: Late effects of polio of concern to Maine people. Maine Nurse 75:5, 8, 1989.

39. Smith DW: Polio and postpolio sequelae: The lived experience. Orthop Nurs 8:24–28, 1989.

40. Speier JL, Owen RR, Knapp M, Canine JK: Occurrence of post-polio sequelae in an epidemic population. In Halstead LS, Wiechers DO (eds): Research and Clinical Aspects of the Late Effects of Poliomyelitis. Birth Defects 23(4):39–48, 1987.

41. Steljes DG, Kryger MH, Kirk BW, et al: Sleep in postpolio syndrome. Chest 98:133–140, 1990.

42. Swan S: Polio survivors find support. Colo Med 81:164, 167, 1984.

43. Tate DG, Forchheimer M, Kirsch N, et al: Prevalence and associated features of depression and psychological distress in polio survivors. Arch Phys Med Rehabil 74:1056–1060, 1993.

44. Twist DJ, Ma DM: Physical therapy management of the patient with post-polio syndrome. Phys Ther 66:1403–1406, 1986.

45. Wiechers DO: Late effects of polio: Historical perspectives. In Halstead LS, Wiechers DO (eds): Research and Clinical Aspects of the Late Effects of Poliomyelitis. Birth Defects 23(4):1–11, 1987.

46. Williams HA, Douglass CS: Nursing implications for post-polio sequelae. Orthop Nurs 5:18–21, 1986.

47. Windebank AJ, Daube JR, Litchy WJ, et al: Late sequelae of paralytic poliomyelitis in Olmsted County, Minnesota. In Halstead LS, Wiechers DO (eds): Research and Clinical Aspects of the Late Effects of Poliomyelitis. Birth Defects 23(4):27–38, 1987.

48. Windebank AJ, Litchy WJ, Daube JR, et al: Late effects of paralytic poliomyelitis in Olmstead County, Minnesota. Neurology 41:501–507, 1991.

49. Winters R: Postpolio syndrome. J Am Acad Nurse Pract 3:69–74, 1991.

50. Young GR: Energy conservation, occupational therapy, and the treatment of post-polio sequelae. Orthopedics 14:1233–1239, 1991.

51. Young GR: Occupational therapy and the postpolio syndrome. Am J Occup Ther 43:97–103, 1989.

12

The Lessons and Legacies of Polio

LAURO S. HALSTEAD, MD

In July 1985, the *New York Times Sunday Magazine* ran an article called the "Painful Legacy of Polio".[4] It described what we now recognize as the late sequelae of polio, or post-polio syndrome, and the point was made that for most of those who had developed paralytic polio many years before, the onset of new symptoms that were related to the old polio was an unexpected experience. Not only were some of the symptoms themselves painful, such as sore muscles and joints, but the whole experience of entering what seemed to be a new and baffling disease process was emotionally and psychologically painful. However, the purpose of this chapter is not to dwell on the physical and psychological pain but rather to step back and view the polio legacy in a larger perspective and to examine some of the lessons that have been learned from dealing with that disease— lessons and legacies that I want to explore on three levels: the individual experience, the social context, and the impact on rehabilitation medicine.

PATHOPHYSIOLOGY OF POLIO

Polio is a unique phenomenon in many ways. It is one of a group of enteroviruses that attacks almost exclusively the anterior horn cells in the spinal cord. Once the virus enters the bloodstream from the intestine and invades the central nervous system, typically 90 to 95% of the anterior **199** horn cells become infected. Some proceed to die, some throw off the virus and return to normal, and some apparently survive the attack but remain impaired in ways that are not clear. Meanwhile, peripherally, a number of complex but fascinating events are occurring: (1) groups of cells that were innervated by motor neurons that have died now become freestanding, fibrillating orphan cells; (2) motor neurons that survived begin to grow additional terminal axon sprouts; and (3) with time, those terminal axon sprouts reinnervate, or adopt, the orphaned muscle fibers. This compensatory process is the one that eventually produced the giant motor units so characteristic of electromyographic (EMG) findings years later in patients who had polio. In addition, the process provides an interesting model of the ways the body responds in some cases to disease—a model that has intriguing implications about how polio has affected people both individually and, on another level, societally.

INDIVIDUAL EXPERIENCE

Beginning on the individual level, consider for a moment someone who develops paralytic poliomyelitis. The disease begins as an acute, febrile illness that over the course of several days results in focal, asymmetric paralysis or possibly even apneic quadriplegia. After emotional recovery from the shock of the initial illness, there follows a period of medical recovery that permits most patients to make some functional gains. And in many instances, patients made spectacular recoveries, going from iron lungs and rocking beds or wheelchairs and braces to using no assistive devices at all. For example, when I had polio, I was 18 years old and had just finished my freshman year in college. I myself made the trip from iron lung to wheelchair to ankle foot orthosis and then to no assistive device in 6 months. Experiences like this left many of us with a number of legacies and lessons that only recently have become clear.

THE LEGACY OF DENIAL

My own experience taught me the mixed blessings of denial. I had recovered and yet did not feel disabled; nor did I grieve. Even though my right arm remained largely paralyzed, I did not think of myself as handicapped. That kind of magical thinking was apparently not unusual among polio patients. In a study of 14 patients and their families that were followed from the onset of illness for up to 2 years, Davis, in *Passage through Crisis*, observed the same attitude repeatedly.[2] For example, all the children who received leg braces while in the hospital did not regard them as a sign of incapacity but rather as proof they were recovering and were ready to go home. They were free of their wheelchairs! What made this kind of remarkable neurologic recovery possible—in addition to surgery and exercise—was the reinnvervation, over a period of 6–12 months, of orphaned muscle cells that rejoined the neuromuscular family by the process of terminal axon sprouting.

To many observers such as family members, the rehabilitation staff, and the patients themselves the recovery sometimes appeared not only complete but miraculous: I could out-leg-wrestle my college roommate, who had enormous thighs from hours of soccer practice. I learned to play squash and tennis better with my left arm than I had with my right before polio. I climbed Mount Fuji in Japan—a journey of over 12,000 feet—on the third anniversary of my polio and left many able-bodied friends puffing away several miles behind. What was I to believe? I knew I wasn't normal. But with the muscles that I had, I could do just about anything I wanted. As a result, I didn't consider myself disabled, and because from the beginning I expected a good recovery, I never went through any serious grieving process. And years later, when new weakness appeared, that denial was still intact, which made understanding and accepting the new changes all the more difficult.

THE LESSON OF EXERCISE AND WORK

Another early lesson most of us learned was the value of exercise. It was a lesson so well learned that it continues to dominate our thinking 30, 40, and 50 years later. For myself, and I know for many others, exercise became an obsession—almost a religious devotion. I made lists of exercises and put them on the wall above my bed. If the therapist said, "Do 10 repetitions twice a day," I would do 20 repetitions three times a day. As my strength returned, I developed a special relationship with my body. I had gained a certain mastery over it and an element of control I had not known before polio. Associated with this sense of mastery and control was the notion that if I worked hard enough, I could accomplish almost anything. Unlike most other neurological diseases and due to the nature of polio, with preserved muscle cells hypertrophying and terminal axon sprouts taking over orphaned muscle cells, it was possible to replace weakness with strength and build strong limbs where atrophic muscle had lain dormant. It was a very viscerel lesson—one that carried over into other aspects of our lives and, I believe, that accounts, in part, for the reason so many polio patients have excelled in their chosen field.

This has, of course, turned out to be both a blessing and a curse. A positive attitude about one's body and the almost supreme hubris about being able to command it to perform any task made many things possible that otherwise might have seemed out of reach. On the other hand, we pushed our bodies when there was pain, when our muscles said no, and when reasonable persons would have rested. That positive attitude also meant that in recent years, when we started to get new weakness, our response was not moderation but to push even harder. Intermittently over the years, as a form of exercise, I used to do a slow jog up six flights of stairs at work. When I first became aware that my legs were growing weaker, my remedy was to do more, not less. I knew what additional exercising had done for me in the past, and therefore, partly because of a stubborn sense of control over my own body, I changed from a slow to a fast jog and increased the number of flights from six to eight. Unfortunately, for me it didn't work. The pathophysiology of my original polio had limits, which became evident only over time. It is now known that one can have clinically normal strength in a muscle with only 45% or 50% of the original nerves supplying that muscle remaining. Thus, while the muscle can function at full strength and appear normal it lacks the normal reserve of the additional neurons that provide backup if anything happens to the functioning nerves. In essence, then, a muscle that is working to its maximum but without reserve is performing the equivalent of a daily marathon: pushing itself to the extreme on a regular basis. In time, there results a depletion of resources with no new compensatory mechanisms to produce more strength. But I now understand why, when patients come to the clinic with new weakness and other symptoms, they believe that once again exercise will be the magic elixir.

THE LESSON OF THE ISOLATING VIRTUES

Our desperate struggle to survive, work hard, and excel led to a series of negative lessons that I believe many of us polios learned, whether we realized it or not. We developed strong denial systems that have kept many of us distanced from the voices of our bodies. We are horrified and outraged at the possibility of being sick again, and we don't want to know that what we worked so hard to achieve might be lost. I believe this helps explain why so many polios are reluctant to seek help when they develop new symptoms. They find it difficult to be vulnerable and are intolerant of weakness in both themselves and others. By walling themselves up, they thus isolate from new disasters and become detached from their own feelings. In addition, the polio experience heightened the prototypic American virtues.

In *The Pursuit of Loneliness,* Slater discusses the isolating virtues that have become so prized in late-20th-century American life, especially by men: so-called virtues such as strength, courage, independence, self-reliance, and hiding your feelings.[6] Many of these virtues are the same ones that enabled us to overcome the challenge of polio and reinforce whatever tendency we had in that direction. But, often unknowingly, we paid a high price. The detachment we learned made it difficult to express emotions and share deeply in relationships. The physical loss sensitized us to other kinds of losses. I developed polio in 1954 but did not experience being disabled until 1982, when I was 46, 28 years later. And it wasn't until several years after that, when I joined a support group and began talking with other polios about my new loss and new pain, that I began to grieve for the body I had lost 30 years earlier. Nowadays, to preserve my weakened leg muscles, I use a motorized scooter at work, take afternoon rest periods that alleviate my fatigue, and, in general, pace my activities from morning till night seven days a week.

I also became aware of how seriously my own sexual-social development had been disrupted. I went from being an able-bodied teenager living away at college to being a quadriparetic son living back at home who needed, for a time, help with toileting, dressing, and bathing. This is clearly not unique to polio, but the rapidity of recovery along with the preservation of bowel, bladder, and sexual function both made it easy to deny much of what had happened and allowed me to pass through a turbulent period of my life without having to confront more directly and honestly my loss and my illness experience.

However, I won't accept all the blame. There were social and medical supports for my denial—beginning right at the top, with Franklin Roosevelt, who was not only a model for recovery but a model for pulling it off with grace, poise, and goodwill. Eleanor and Franklin were household heroes long before I had polio, but then when I developed his illness, he took on special significance. We know now, however, through Gallagher's *FDR's Splendid Deception,* that FDR was much more like us than we realized—particularly in his efforts to deny his disability.[3]

THE LEGACY OF FEELING IMMORTAL AND BEING CHOSEN

Another legacy is our sense of immortality and being chosen to be tested. For infants and children too young to be aware of what was going on, I believe this was an attitude shared by both parents and staff. For myself at 18, even though for a while I was in an iron lung, I had the simple faith that I would survive. And not only would I survive, but I would regain my health quickly—in a week or two at most! I realize part of such thinking is absolutely normal on the part of any healthy teenager suddenly rendered desperately ill regardless of the disease. But part of it, I believe, was also the knowledge that most polios did recover—some of them so completely it was difficult to know they were disabled. In addition, the hospital where I was recovering was full of other polios—and the mood among the patients and staff was extraordinarily positive and hopeful—unlike in any hospital units I have ever seen since. Yet, that positive spirit had negative moral implications. Good people got better; bad people did not improve; and some even died. This message taught people to survive and deny. Nothing less was acceptable.

Other parts of this legacy have to do with messages we were told. Polio children were sometimes led to believe their illness was a God-given challenge. How else can we explain a disease that appeared to strike randomly, a disease that hit without warning, when you were healthy, and that you did nothing to bring on? A child struck by a car because of failing to look both ways before crossing the street is understandable; a child paralyzed during the night while asleep is an act of God. "God gives us only what we can handle," the saying goes; "God gives the heaviest crosses to the ones he loves the best," is another. The real message, however, is, "You're special. Be strong. Don't cry. Make Mama proud. Show God that he was right." No wonder the average level of education among polios is said to be higher than that of the general population. And is it any wonder that the rate of employment among polio survivors is reported to be four times the rate of the disabled population at large? The potential for motor recovery is unlike that of most other neuromuscular diseases and when combined with a sense of "special mission"—wherever that idea came from—the results could be spectacular. Add to this a society that was supportive if not at times indulgent, and you had polio patients, who felt special, even chosen.

SOCIAL CONTEXT

LEGACY OF THE FORGOTTEN DISEASE

The first social legacy is that polio the disease, along with its survivors, has been forgotten. It's interesting to speculate why and how this occurred. Even though the major polio epidemics of the 1930s, '40s, and '50s were becoming larger and larger, the overall mortality rate (approximately 12%) was particularly high compared to some of the major killers during the same period, such as tuberculosis, heart disease, and cancer. So, numbers alone didn't make polio an important disease. As Davis says, "Epidemiological statistics alone cannot account for the awe and dread with which polio had come to be regarded or for the very special consideration and mass sympathy extended to its victims."[2] Polio often hit children, and the sight of children with braces and wheelchairs broke America's heart.

Those of you who remember that time can recall the fear and hysteria. No one knew who might be struck down next, which created a feeling of ambivalence in our society. There was a love-hate relationship with polio. As Sontag writes in *Illness as Metaphor*, "Any disease that is treated as a mystery and acutely enough feared will be felt to be morally, if not literally, contagious."[8] On one hand, there were extraordinary dread of infection, fear of paralysis and death, and the more subtle underlying sense of moral vulnerability; on the other hand, for those who survived, there was a tendency to romanticize the survivor, and in fact, for a time, entire communities became large support groups.

Many Americans over the age of 40 know of individuals who developed polio, then began to recover; before long, the whole community was rallying around. Pictures were in the newspapers, and there were frequent follow-up stories—sometimes promising a bit more recovery than had actually occurred. In many locales, mothers were identified as constituting the primary workforce to establish a door-to-door, volunteer fund-raising campaign. This created the impact of a crusade: the mothers' crusade, or, as the March of Dimes later phrased it, the "Mothers' March against Polio." It was a clever piece of merchandising and reflected the first time mothers and their emotional instincts to save and preserve the family were exploited on the behalf of science or, more accurately, on behalf of a fundraising organization. Thus, as a society, we used the suffering of polio patients and the guilt of those who survived untouched to create a fabulously wealthy industry. Within a few years, the March of Dimes grew to be a national organization that reached into virtually every community, becoming the most successful charitable organization in history.

Speaking of the impact of the March of Dimes, Davis wrote, "It is not surprising, therefore, that of the many critical diseases which afflict man, polio had come to occupy a pre-eminent and according to some, an exaggerated place in the awareness, sympathy and philanthropy of the American people. It was regarded as a powerful symbol of blind, devastating and uncontrolled misfortune whose victims were especially entitled to the support and good will of the community."[2]

The legacy of that development is mixed. Some of the money was used for direct patient services: I in fact was a beneficiary of money raised by my mother and her friends, for all of my hospital charges were automatically paid by the March of Dimes, as were charges for my outpatient therapy and any other associated expenses. This was one of the great benefits given to the individual by the March of Dimes. But there was also a hidden side to how the funds were used. Money began to dictate diagnosis. Patients who presented to a hospital—especially indigent patients—with an unclear diagnosis but with several symptoms suggestive of polio or during the midst of a polio epidemic, frequently were admitted with a firm diagnosis of polio because it guaranteed that both the hospital and the doctor would be paid and those patients' needs met.

As a result, many people today who never actually had polio believe they had the disease and can often show hospital records to prove it. This is unfortunate for several reasons. First, it falsely inflates the number of people who claim they had polio, which distorts any efforts to determine the true prevalence of the number of survivors, and second, it creates unnecessary confusion and hardship among patients who are experiencing post-polio-like symptoms and mistakenly believe some of them with extraordinary conviction) they are suffering from the late effects of polio. Occasionally, some of these individuals have carried their polio label with them for a lifetime and used it to explain all sorts of ills as well as why their lives have never been as fulfilled as they had hoped.

In addition to educating the public and paying for health services, the March of Dimes used its money to support research. In 1955, Salk's inactivated vaccine was introduced. Newsreel footage from those days shows the banner headline: "Polio Conquered." It had been another war and we had won. American technology had scored another knockout. In small towns all across America, there were parades with marching bands and big signs proclaiming "Victory over Polio." There was a cure for polio, but it wasn't for those who had it. *The victory was for those who would never get it.*

Thus, the impact on the American psyche was the *feeling* that polio had been conquered. As a result, polio slowly dropped out of the national consciousness by slipping off the national agenda. Unlike other countries were March of Dimes–type organizations continued to work with polio survivors, the American March of Dimes changed its name and its corporate identity and in the early 1960s became the Birth Defects Foundation. There were no more campaigns for the heroic survivors of polio. There was no longer a national organization or a national support group. There were not even local support groups.

There was no new research and only a few publications. Medically, polio was beginning a historical oddity. In medical schools, it existed as an interesting case study of the wonders of modern technology and as an important disease of note in the Third World. And clinical descriptions in standard medical textbooks were, we now know, often misleading. As late as 1982, in Krusen's *Handbook of Physical Medicine and Rehabilitation,* polio was still classified as a *static* motor unit disease, meaning, no late phase of new weakness or motor neuron deterioration was recognized.[5]

Because there was very little in the medical literature about late neurological changes, for most health practitioners that possibility did not exist. And social silence supported both the individual denial and the professional ignorance. Thus, the initial response made by friends, family members, and health professionals to new health problems among polio survivors was that nothing was wrong. How could it be? Polio had been conquered. Polio was a static disease. You've done well all these years, so why should anything change? These were the messages we heard. When the symptoms would not go away, however, and we became persistent, the most common responses then were "It's all in your head," or "You're under a lot of stress," or "You're going through a midlife crisis."

As we now know, polio survivors were experiencing something that occurs less and less commonly in medicine—they were dealing with a new cluster of symptoms that had no name, and without a name there was not a disease. The history of medicine is the history of taxonomy. When malaria was believed to be due to swamp fog, medicine gave it a name by calling it miasma. Having a name implied a cause and opened up the possibility of treatment and even a cure. But in a sophisticated era, when many diseases had been totally eliminated with vaccines, what was there new to learn? In effect, post-polio syndrome for a period of time was an orphan disease. No name, no organization, and no funding agency to adopt it.

THE LEGACY OF DISABILITY COMMERCIALIZATION

Another social legacy was the development of the poster child by the March of Dimes. It was an ingenious fund-raising technique and so successful that it has been adopted to this day by every other fund-raising organization that deals with disabled children. Unfortunately, however, it helped initiate and perpetuate the commercialization of disability. And in so doing, it has helped create and then reinforce many of the negative stereotypes about disability. It also marked the beginning of large fundraising organizations' trying to define how we perceive and think about disability. Naturally, only the right kids could be chosen to be poster children. So, inevitably there were competitions. Kids couldn't be too sick, say, in an iron lung, or too well, say, with no visible deformity. They had to be cute but with an obvious need and showing a lot of grit. But above all, they couldn't offend. The best candidates were usually little girls with winning smiles and shiny, long leg braces. The photos demonstrated the poster child's obvious needs and also made it clear she was a fighter who would do even better with your generous contribution.[7]

As it turned out, the poster kids became media stars one moment and then forgotten kids with chronic illnesses the next. And now, 30 years later, many of these same individuals are developing new health problems related to their old polio, but the March of Dimes has abandoned them.

Another legacy of the March of Dimes was to help create a climate in which individual disease entities began competing with each other for limited resources. Over the years, this has led to a proliferation of disease-specific charity groups and the Americanization of disability research and services. I don't believe the unplanned capitalistic, free market approach has served the disability community well, however. It has led to the fragmentation of disability groups—all competing for the same resources— and to a redundancy of bureaucracy and effort that have all too often resulted in the isolation of individuals and groups and the squandering of precious assets by combating each other instead of the disease.

The exploitation of children to raise money continues to this day by means of such events as the Muscular Dystrophy Labor Day Telethon with Jerry Lewis and Jerry's kids. Although the Mother's March is still used by the Birth Defects Foundation, it has been largely replaced by a more successful strategy of national walkathons that pits corporation against corporation so that Team Xerox tries to outdo Team Shell. All of which may be a great way to raise money and perhaps raise someone's consciousness, but it is a hell of a way to decide health care priorities or to entice people into paying their fair share. I don't mean to imply that the March of Dimes fund raising of 30 and 40 years ago is responsible for our patchwork approach to disability today, but it did reinforce the American ideal of individual initiative as a way of dealing with serious health problems.

THE LEGACY OF LOCAL SUPPORT GROUPS

And now the cycle is beginning anew. Because there is no national organization, we are having to rediscover our own power, our own needs, and each other. Over the years, with a few exceptions, I was careful to avoid other polios and would never have belonged to a polio survivor organization. After all, I had overcome polio and didn't want to be identified with a disability group. But, when I began to have new health problems related to my polio, I changed my mind. And apparently the same thing was true for thousands of other polio survivors.

Unfortunately, this time around, there are a number of strikes against us. There are no national epidemics; there are no adorable poster kids to create public sympathy; many of the people who want to take action are having health problems and don't have the energy to put into a new organization; and there are innumerable well-organized, highly publicized groups representing other health care problems that compete for the available dollars. However, the picture is not entirely bleak.

In the past few years, a unique and quintessentially American phenomenon has emerged. In the presence of a vacuum, people stepped in. Rather than wait for government, the rehabilitation profession, or someone else to take action, polio survivors all over the country began to realize that if something were to be done, they would have to do it themselves. And that is how the post-polio support group movement came into being, which currently numbers more than 300 organizations. The groups have slowly begun to develop a power base of their own, which in turn has led to the beginnings of a national organization and social movement to pressure funding agencies and initiate new research

IMPACT ON REHABILITATION MEDICINE

THE LEGACY OF POLIO AND REHABILITATION MEDICINE

Polio and rehabilitation have clearly been good for each other. The big epidemics created a health care crisis that other specialties were not equipped to handle. Pediatricians, internists, and general practitioners usually made the diagnosis and guided their patients through the acute phase, and orthopedists followed up in ensuing years with reconstructive surgery. But in the meantime, there was a need for a specialty that could address all the fragmented pieces of care over an extended period of time and provide a holistic, integrated perspective. There was a need for a specialty that concerned itself with such diverse issues as functional performance, kinesiology, muscle physiology, orthotics, bowel and bladder function, respiratory physiology, vocational training, psychological adjustment, and family needs. And there was a need for a speciality that valued the importance of working together with allied health professionals in a team setting. Although practitioners in the fledgling field of physiatry or physical medicine and rehabilitation (rehabilitation medicine, for short) couldn't address all these needs at the outset, in many ways the multiple requirements of polio patients helped challenge the emerging specialty to expand and grow and ultimately to define itself. For these reasons, polio was the prototypic disease of rehabilitation medicine, and to treat polio patients properly required specialized facilities, staff, and programs. Many of the major rehabilitation programs around the country began as polio centers, and when acute polio disappeared many of these centers applied their expertise to an expanded group of chronic and disabling conditions in both children and adults. Today, post-polio clinics are centers for learning the new skills and lessons of how best to care for persons aging with a disability.

THE LEGACY OF SPECIALIZED CARE

The management of polio patients required a broad spectrum of care. On one end were patients who had mild paralysis and thus could participate in fairly vigorous therapy almost from the time of admission. The major concern for many of these patients was to modulate their zeal by preventing them from exercising too hard and too fast. While not widely appreciated, overuse weakness among polios was a distinct phenomenon described in the medical literature as early as 1958 by Bennett and Knowlton.[1]

On the other end of the spectrum of polio patients were those who developed respiratory failure as part of their acute illness. By necessity, physicians and allied health personnel quickly become proficient in the management of these patients as well. When the patient could tolerate it, therapists initiated daily treatments while the patient was still in the iron lung. Frequently, because of the large number of ventilator patients and the shortage of staff—especially of nursing staff at night—a group of ventilator patients were clustered together in one area. Apparently, that kind of clustering of very sick patients gave birth to the intensive care unit, which was later adopted for many other kinds of patients by general hospitals.

While much of the expertise and comfort in dealing with the acutely ill patient has been lost in rehabilitation hospitals, some of it has been preserved in those centers that manage high-spinal-cord-injured apneic quadriplegics. Of course, the expertise and comfort gained in managing complicated polio patients were not limited to treating acute medical problems: it extended throughout the hospital wherever patients were treated and into the postdischarge efforts to reintegrate people into the community and find meaningful employment. Imagine! Ventilator-dependent patients in competitive employment. Now that's an excellent example of the specialized medical care that is made possible by a team of rehabilitation professionals, and it's a direct legacy of the lessons learned managing respiratory polio patients.

THE LEGACY OF HOSPITAL-BASED TREATMENT

As I indicated earlier, some of the legacies from the polio era have resulted in mixed blessings. Rehabilitation has always prided itself in its provision of comprehensive, coordinated care that involves multiple disciplines. Because of the complexity and acuteness of disease in many of the polio patients, it was natural that a large proportion of such patients' initial care was provided in the hospital. With time, this evolved into a tradition for treating other diseases as well—a tradition wherein the majority of services were hospital based and delivered in a single setting. While this was both convenient for the staff and cost-efficient for a time, it also had the undesirable—and perhaps largely unexpected—effect of creating a mind-set about the nature and scope of rehabilitation services as well as where they could be provided. Underlying this was the more subtle issue of control. As long as services were hospital based, patients could be more easily controlled by the hospital professionals, which ironically tended to foster a form of dependency on the very persons that such professionals were encouraging to be more independent.

Much of that has changed in recent years, of course, partly due to the disability rights and independent living movements, partly due to a more sophisticated and flexible vision of rehabilitation, and partly due to the financing realities of rehabilitation care today.

THE LEGACY OF BEING FORGOTTEN

The legacy of being forgotten is related to the previous one of hospital-based orientation. For many polio patients, including myself, being discharged from the hospital marked the end of a formal rehabilitation program. It's true I continued to exercise on my own and observed the recommendations made during my hospital stay, but I never received a single follow-up letter or questionnaire and was never given an appointment for a checkup in the clinic of either hospital where I had been treated. I know this wasn't true of every rehabilitation center, but from patients I have talked to and examined in recent years, I get the impression this occurred more often than not. When follow-up did occur, it tended to be a single service, such as a brace check, and only infrequently included a comprehensive reevaluation.

Nor do I believe the hospitals were entirely to blame. I myself could have taken the initiative, but from what I've said earlier, in my case—and I believe it was true for others was well—the overwhelming urge was to put the experience behind me. Returning to the hospital—even as a visitor— would have reminded me of an illness I wanted to forget and one I thought I had conquered. Therefore, just perhaps, another visit would have reminded me that I really was disabled.

Because I and thousands like me did not return to hospitals over the years, I believe both the hospitals (and indirectly the field of rehabilitation) and the polio survivors were cheated. Hospitals lost a marvelous opportunity to track the neurological and functional course of polio, which might have given them advance warning about some of the deterioration that caught so many of us by surprise. Follow-up might also have helped create a knowledge base that could have been applied as part of a prevention program to minimize, delay, or even avoid the late neurologic changes. Clearly, however, this is a lesson that has been learned, because one need only look at the aggressive follow-up programs for spinal-cord-injured patients and other disability groups that exist at most rehabilitation hospitals today.

In addition to failing to create a knowledge base that might have helped individual polio survivors cope better, the field of rehabilitation, in a larger sense, I believe, also failed society. Through their various professional organizations, rehabilitation staffs communicate new knowledge and keep other health professionals, consumers, and society at large educated and informed. In fact, it is just this process that helps shape the agenda for future services, training, and research.

However, in the absence of new information, old polio problems did not get updated and were not even included on new agendas. This is exactly what happened to polio through the 1960s, 70s, and early 80s. Fortunately, the situation has begun to change, but there remains a lot of work to be done on behalf of the thousands of survivors still alive today.

Paradoxically, I believe many of these survivors might be in a position to benefit rehabilitation. Many have been successful in their chosen professions, and many are in the public eye. Providing them with an ongoing forum in which they could be involved in their local rehabilitation centers, promoting not only the cause of polio but rehabilitation causes in general, might be a way of mobilizing an enormous untapped reservoir of goodwill and possible financial support.

THE LESSON OF AGING WITH A DISABILITY

Here is an important lesson that has formed as a result of the recent attention focused on the health problems of the polio population. Even if there were no neurologic changes, there would inevitably be aches and pains of muscles and joints and a gradual slowing down due to wear and tear, for a wounded organ never performs as well as an intact one. Trieschmann, in *Aging with a Disability*, reminds us that members of the polio population constitute the first group that benefited from rehabilitation in large numbers and are now reaching the time of life when many of its members are experiencing the effects of aging.[9] The point she makes so eloquently is that all of us who are physically disabled undergo double jeopardy. It is not a simple additive effect. Frequently, polio survivors have managed to move through life at a great cost in energy and by performing a kind of balancing act: using preserved muscles to the maximum and often in ways that were never intended. Aging has the effect of disrupting that balance and exacting a price far greater than when it occurs in an intact person. And in turn, the underlying disability appears to accelerate and possibly magnify the usual effects of aging. In the presence of new neurologic losses, the consequences can be devastating.

To the extent that polio survivors have been neglected by their old rehabilitation hospitals and to the extent that they have by choice elected to avoid contact with health professionals, their recent and rather sudden reappearance in doctors' office and polio clinic around the country has served to heighten the impact of this final lesson: don't neglect yourself as you age and don't let yourself be neglected. It is a lesson that is being eagerly and quickly applied to other population groups as well, notably, the spinal cord injured. Even in the absence of new health problems and even in persons in their 20s, 30s, and 40s, it's not too early to begin applying some of the common-sense approaches to aging that are being advocated for everyone, such as improved nutrition, achieving ideal body weight, regular and sensible exercise, and frequent checkups.

CONCLUSION

During the mid-1980s, there was considerable speculation about the exact number of polio survivors in the United States. Clearly, it is an important piece of information to have and is crucial in a determination of the size of the commitment made in addressing polio survivors' needs. Based on an informal survey conducted in 1977 by the National Center for Health Statistics, approximately 300,000 persons in the United States were identified who had residual paralysis from polio.

However, because renewed interest in the fate of the polio population in the 80s, a formal survey on polio survivors was included in the 1987 National Health Interview Survey.[10] The preliminary analyses of this study are important and make fascinating reading. Based on probability sampling, it is estimated there are 1.6 million people in the United States who were told by a physician or other health professional they had polio. Of these, 640,000 experienced paralysis associated with their polio. Although it is not clear how many have residual paralysis, the group of 640,000 who experienced paralysis at the time of their polio represents the population at risk for developing long-term sequelae. Potentially this means more than twice as many polio survivors who might require services as we originally thought. For me personally, it means twice as many comrades in arms; for society, it means considerably more resources will need to be committed to helping those with new health problems. For those of us who practice in rehabilitation, it means more work and a far greater challenge in dealing with the ongoing legacy of polio than we realized.

REFERENCES

1. Bennett RL, Knowlton GC: Overwork weakness in partially denervated muscle. Clin Orthop 12:22–49, 1958.
2. Davis F. Passage through Crisis. New York, The Bobbs Merrill Co., 1963.
3. Gallagher HG: FDR's Splendid Deception. Arlington,VA, Vandamere Press, 1994.
4. Horowitz J: The Painful Legacy of Polio. New York Times Sunday Magazine, July 5, 1985.
5. Johnson EW, Alexander MA: Management of motor unit disease. In Krusen F (ed): Handbook of Physical Medicine and Rehabilitation. Philadelphia, W.B. Saunders, 1982.
6. Slater PE: The Pursuit of Loneliness: American Culture at the Breaking Point. Boston, Beacon Press, 1970.
7. Smith JS: Patenting the Sun: Polio and the Salk Vaccine. New York, Morrow, 1990.
8. Sontag S: Illness as Metaphor. New York, Farrar, Straus and Giroux, 1977.
9. Trieschmann R: Aging with a Disability. New York, Demos, 1987.
10. Parsons PE: [Letter]. N Engl J Med 325:1108, 1991.

13

Growing Old with Polio: A Personal Perspective

HUGH GREGORY GALLAGHER

"I'll rack thee with old cramps,
Fill all thy bones with aches, make thee roar
That beasts shall tremble at thy din."
—Prospero's curse of Caliban
Shakespeare, *The Tempest*

I am a person with quadriplegic polio and a member of the first large-scale generation of those seriously paralyzed by polio to survive into old age. Thanks to antibiotics, advancements in medical care, orthotics, and good luck, I'm still here. I have lived with my disability—independent and

The author is a writer and consultant based in Washington, D.C. In 1952, at the age of 19, he contracted a severe case of spinal and bulbar poliomyelitis. Completely paralyzed during the acute stage of his illness, Gallagher was in an iron lung for 6 weeks, in the hospital for 12 months, and in rehabilitation at Warm Springs, Georgia, for an additional 9 months. Over many months of physical therapy, he recovered partial, yet functional, use of his shoulders, arms, and hands. His trunk and leg muscles remain paralyzed. At Warm Springs, Gallagher's scapulae were stabilized by means of a fasciotomy, thereby improving the function of his arms and shoulder muscles. Gallagher has lived independently and alone for over 40 years; he uses an electric wheelchair, drives his own car, and is self-supporting.

self-supporting—for more than 40 years. And now, like many others, I find my polio-ravaged muscles are developing new weakness, new cramps, new aches; my energy and endurance are leaching away.

Whatever the cause of this—and there are conflicting theories—I must live with it. This is my problem and the subject of this chapter. How do I maintain the quality of my life as I age?

How to deal with aging has been a search older than Hippocrates. The problems faced by persons aging with polio are not different in kind from those of the aging able-bodied, but they *are* different—very different—in degree. Age comes earlier, with greater impact to those with polio. What is no more than annoying to the aging able-bodied can be totally disabling to the aging person with polio.

Everybody is different: everyone has different problems and different solutions. The problems have common threads, and perhaps some of my own experiences will be helpful to other people with polio (and their health providers) as they wrestle with their own unique problems.

Here are five aspects of dealing with the late effects of polio that I have found to be of particular importance to those aging with Polio—at least, to my aging with polio: the medical profession, economics, engineering, psychological, and philosophical.

THE MEDICAL PROFESSION

Doctors today know little about polio. With the exception of the older generation of physicians, now retiring from practice, and certain specialists in physical medicine, most of today's physicians have never seen an active case. The late effects of polio, their impact on the aging process, and what is now generally called post-polio syndrome—these things often go unrecognized and misdiagnosed. I know people with polio who have been treated for conditions they did not have, as well as others who have been told erroneously that their complaints were psychological in origin and that relief should be sought in psychotherapy.

I believe today's persons with polio, to the extent possible, should act as their own chief doctor. Only *I* know what it takes for me to remain functional in my daily living. Only *I* know what impact bed rest has and what impact a hospital stay can have on my functional ability and personal esteem. Only *I* know, after many years of experience, the sort of reactions that various medications can have on my body. Only *I* know how to monitor myself closely. Only *I* have developed an early warning system to detect and deal with problems before they become major.

I do not mean that I know more about medicine then does my physician. Not at all. I know more about *me*. When I consult my doctors, they bring to the conference their knowledge of medicine, and I bring my knowledge of my paralyzed body. Together, we analyze what is wrong, what treatment is advisable, and what impact that treatment is likely to have on the problem and on my ability to function independently.

I have found that once this approach is explained, physicians accept its premise and appreciate it. Many find it a heavy burden to be the God-like father-physician, making life or death decisions for compliant, all-trusting patients. I have found that responsible physicians are willing—even relieved—to share some of that burden. If your doctor does not accept such an approach, find another doctor.

The care and maintenance of an aging, severely paralyzed polio body is not a simple business. I have made a list of the things I do on a daily basis (Table 1). The regimen sounds fairly onerous, but it is made easier by daily repetition.

TABLE 1. Daily Monitoring of an Independent-Living Quadriplegic Polio

1. Sleep on stomach with legs extended to keep hamstrings from tightening.
2. Inspect buttocks for pressure points; massage with moisturizer.
3. Inspect legs and feet for swelling and fluid retention; take diuretic as needed.
4. Inspect toes and legs for cracks, cuts, etc.; apply topical antibiotic as needed.
5. Monitor urine flow; be on guard for urine retention.
6. Watch for fungus infections in crotch area, particularly in hot weather.
7. Make sure bowels are regular; be on guard against constipation and impaction.
8. Use moleskin and topical antibiotic as needed on skin abrasions caused by back brace/corset.
9. Perform deep breathing exercises throughout the day to keep weak lungs in optimal condition.
10. Exercise and stretch arms and shoulders, using a broomstick.
11. Take 10 mg methyltestosterone daily for maintenance of muscle strength and tone.
12. Treat facial acne caused by methyltestosterone with Retin A and topical antibiotic as needed.
13. Follow a low-fat, low-calorie diet; keep weight as low as possible to minimize muscle strain in making transfers.
14. Take high-level vitamin and mineral dietary supplements to guard against possible deficiencies caused by low level of food intake.
15. Have weekly massage, stretching, and exercise sessions.

ECONOMICS

My muscle power and endurance are as coins in my purse: I have only so many and they will buy only so much. I must live within my means, and to do this I have to economize: what do I want to buy and how can I buy it for the least possible cost? In terms of muscle power and endurance, I can still pretty much go wherever I used to and do pretty much what I used to—but not as easily and not as often. I must assign priorities and ration my activities. I shop around and plan ahead.

Growing old with polio is a matter of economics: cost/benefit analysis. How much expenditure of limited energy for how much satisfaction. Minimize the exertion; maximize the pleasure.

Polio-weakened muscles have a finite, lifetime limit. I know people with polio who refuse to accommodate their lifestyle to their weakening muscle condition. They function on willpower, forcing their muscles, without regard to pain or spasm, to do their daily duty as they have in times past. This is like using up your IRA retirement account too soon before you are dead. It can be a desperate game. One such person I know of, after years of "walking" on willpower alone, committed suicide rather than use a wheelchair. Others grumble a lot but adjust as they move from braces to a wheelchair, or, like me, from a manual chair to an electric.

In my own case, I can no longer work full-time in an office environment. I work part-time at home and live more modestly. I am poorer, but it seems to me, my life is richer.

ENGINEERING

Most of us with polio have struggled throughout our lives to be as independent and self-reliant as possible. Now, after all these years, when we find we must accept more help, we feel a real sense of failure: we have fought the good fight—and lost it.

In my own case, for many years I refused to admit that I needed an electric wheelchair. In spite of aches, increasing fatigue, and an ever-narrowing range of mobility, I was determined to tough it out with my manual chair. Finally, when I could tough no longer, when I was forced to transfer to an electric, I was surprised by how greatly the quality and independence of my life improved. Better equipment makes for better living.

Over the years there have been significant improvements in orthotics, equipment, electronics, public attitudes, and accessibility. All of the following have improved the quality of life of disabled people: lightweight braces; practical, even portable, electric wheelchairs; dependable van lifts; personal computers; improved transportation practices and access for the traveling disabled; drive-in automatic teller machines; telephone grocery services; and cable TV.

These things and many more are right at hand to make things easier for the ingenious quadriplegic. For those with major paralysis, it takes the inventiveness of a Rube Goldberg and the skill of an engineer if they are to maximize functional ability. There is usually a way—one way or another—to get something done.

The problem of severely limited muscle power and the resulting restrictions on mobility can be analyzed in terms of Newtonian physics: mass, inertia, and the application of force. A knowledge of the uses of leverage, pivot points, inclined planes, and centers of gravity makes them invaluable tools. I am fortunate to have had training in the principles of static and dynamic mechanics. These have stood me in good stead as I analyze how to get me—and by body—from A to B and back again. Though this intellectual approach has indeed been most helpful, I do not mean to diminish the value of plain intuition. Most of us wheelchair users, over the years, develop a pretty accurate intuitive understanding of what will work and what will not.

The Rube Goldberg aspect is using what is at hand to do what must be done. I need to get something from the high shelf in the closet, so I claw it down with a straightened-out coat-hanger. I carry an ordinary ice bag with me at all times—an unobtrusive, portable urinal. An old piece of cowhide—slick on one side, rough on the other—serves as a portable "slide board." A stick with an eggcup on its end allows me, after I have transferred myself into my car, to steer my electric wheelchair far enough away from the car to close the door.

I get a nice sense of satisfaction when I figure out how to do something that I could not do before. This satisfaction is familiar to all polio survivors.

PSYCHOLOGY

My rehabilitation at Warm Springs, Georgia, was a remarkably positive experience. There was a contagious can-do enthusiasm there, not unlike the enthusiasm of a football team on a winning streak. We were *pumped.*

We encouraged ourselves in the denial of the extent of our impairment. Unwittingly, we taught ourselves to hide it and work like hell to overcome it. With polio, this approach was remarkably effective. Polio is not a progressive condition. Maximum paralysis occurs at the height of the critical stage of the disease; with informed exercise and care, over a period of months and years, the paralyzed muscles regain—and *retain*—a significant degree of strength and function. At Warm Springs, we translated this into "work hard, push the limit, and you can make your muscles do what you tell them to."

For me, this approach worked well for many years. I used my willpower to drive my severely limited muscle power. Now I find the game has an end point. No matter how much willpower is applied, my muscles are worn out. They can no longer do what they used to—and when they do what they still can do, it is only with pain and vast fatigue.

And here I confront the central enigma of polio: If I give up and let other people do for me the things I usually do for myself, my muscles rest and I feel fine. But then, in a very short period of time, I lose what remaining strength I have left and—soon enough—I can no longer do anything for myself at all. And then I don't feel fine at all. So there is no alternative: use it or lose it. And so I soldier on, all aches—like Caliban.

There was another, rather more complicated aspect to rehabilitation at Warm Springs. This was a direct legacy of Warm Springs' founder, Franklin Delano Roosevelt.[1] We were encouraged; we encouraged each other to maintain a heroic charade. We convinced ourselves that, regarding our disability, we never thought about it, and we were never bothered by it; we could, and we would, do anything an able-bodied person did—or die in the attempt.

And die we almost did. As the body rebelled, the fake facade became harder, ultimately impossible to maintain. And yet—I was loath to let it go. So much of my pride, persona, and self-image was invested in this heroic charade. It was the way I saw myself; it was my shield; with it I was invulnerable. Without it, what was I?

And the answer was hard to come by: without the charade, I was just human. It is, after all, superhuman to be always indomitable in the face of all events, to persevere without complaint no matter what. This is far more exhausting than mere physical fatigue. Not only is it superhuman; it is pointless. After all these years, I have earned the right to be human, to complain, and if warranted, to cry out with Caliban, "That beasts shall tremble at thy din."

I have found it something like a liberation at last to be honest to oneself and one's world. If the charade was a shield, it was also a wall. It kept me from sharing my feelings with other people—it isolated me from them. That is too bad because I had much to share with them and much support to gain from them.

PHILOSOPHY

It seems to me that people with polio have an advantage over the able-bodied when it comes to aging. Polios know things the able-bodied do not. They have, perhaps, a certain wisdom. Many of us have looked death in the eye. From our childhood, we have known what it is to lose control, to be helpless, to suffer pain, to be terrified. And yet—as William Faulkner put it—not merely to endure but to prevail.

And now, post-polio syndrome provides a refresher course. This knowledge of ours—painfully learned—gives a unique perspective on aging. It brings us both advantages and serious responsibility.

The advantages are of two types. The restrictions imposed by age are not new to us. We already know how to live with limited mobility, limited energy, and chronic pain. We do not confuse the quality of our life with the quality of our tennis game. We know that happiness is not dependent on activity, nor is value measured by tennis trophies. A meaningful life may be hampered by—but need not be defined by—pain or disability.

The second advantage comes from our familiarity with death. We know death; it is not the enemy it is to able-bodied people. Death is the end, but that is all it is. We know, better than most, that we need not panic over our own mortality. As we get older, as our polio-frail muscles give out, we are reminded again—and forcefully—how fragile as thing is well-being. Our understanding of the ever presence of death means that we do not defer living. More than most, we live in the now.

It is, as I see it, our responsibility to share this specialized knowledge of ours with able-bodied friends and family as they grow old.

Today, America is obsessed with youth and fitness. In television sitcoms, commercials, and mail order catalogs, everyone is trim, slim, and young. It is popularly taken as a matter of fact that proper diet and regular exercise guarantee well-being. The miracles of modern medicine, glowingly reported in the media, are popularly held to promise a long and youthful life.

As a result, when decrepitude, disease, and death come—as inevitably they do—they come as a surprise. It is then that the able-bodied turn to us. And it is then our responsibility to help them as they have helped us with our disability over all these years.

Susan Sontag has written, "Everyone who is born holds dual citizenship in the kingdom of the well and the kingdom of the sick." Persons with polio can serve as guides to their families and friends as it becomes others' turn to pass through the kingdom of the sick.

It is not easy for a person to understand the pain and fear of others and to reach out to them. Yet now, it seems to me, we with polio find ourselves in a position to do just that. This is our gift, if we will use it. By so doing, we help others and we enrich and make more meaningful our own lives.

REFERENCE

1. Gallagher HG: *FDR's Splendid Deception.* Arlington, VA, Vandamere Press, 1994.

Index

Page numbers in **boldface** indicate complete chapters.

223